Strategic Healthcare Management

Applying the Lessons of Today's
Top Management Experts to
the Business of Managed Care

Ira Studin

A Healthcare 2000 Publication

 IRWIN
Professional Publishing®
Burr Ridge, Illinois
New York, New York

A **2000** *PUBLICATION*

ISBN 1-55738-631-5

Printed in the United States of America

BB

1 2 3 4 5 6 7 8 9 0

JB

For Gail, Sara, and Zachary

with love

"Unless structure follows strategy, inefficiency results."

— Alfred Chandler

Table of Contents

Acknowledgements

Much of what I have learned about the healthcare industry derives from over seven years of working with Barbara Grenell and Debbie Brandel at Preferred Health Strategies. Thanks for the good times. Thanks to David Assael, Burt Deixler, Mark Gottdiener, Bob Handler, John Petterson, Howard Reiss, and Ed Spiro, who, in different ways, helped me as only good friends can. Thanks as well to Jamie Kasman for his assistance with a number of graphics. And thanks to Kristine Rynne, of Irwin, for believing in the entire project.

I could not have written this book were it not for the first-class education I received from three world-class institutions: Colgate University; the University of California, San Diego (UCSD); and the University of California, Los Angeles (UCLA). Though their good counsel was provided years ago, I benefited enormously from from three advisors extraordinaire: Arnold Sio at Colgate; Joseph Gusfield at UCSD; and Paul Torrens at UCLA.

Long ago, my parents instilled in me a healthy respect for learning, high ideals, and a deep and abiding sense of craft. I thank you both. Thanks to two great sisters—Cindi Berger and Jan Studin; and three aunts and uncles—Ellen and Seymour Studin, Danny and Millie Rothenberg, and Babe and Hal Adams—all supportive in their own way. To Babe and Hal, thank you for showing me your way of looking, of appreciating, and of providing perspective.

Ideas, I believe, are socially determined. Fortunately, the social circumstances affecting me the most stem from my wife Gail and our two children, Sara and Zachary. Gail, your respect for my efforts provided a continuous source of comfort and your encouragement, a special kind of energy. Sara, thank you for regularly reminding me I am an author. Zachary, thank you for always being interested and asking about my progress. I don't know whether the time taken from each of you can ever be repaid, but please know that you each brought out the very best I could bring to this project. Beyond that, "you know what I have to say."

Introduction

Not long ago, I met with a senior physician on the faculty practice of a prominent medical school, one of the temples of American medicine. At the time, I was interviewing him as part of a consulting engagement. All of a sudden, he got out of his chair, walked to his desk, and tossed a letter at me in disgust. The letter, from the school's hospital, said his health insurance was being terminated. He was panicked and did not know what to do. The irony of that situation did not escape me.

We live in an age where the reach of medical science is unparalleled and frustration with healthcare delivery trickles down to every segment of society. The contrast between the capabilities of medical science and the limitations of medical organization may well be the imprimatur of American medicine in the current age.

Healthcare in the United States is a trillion dollar industry that resists the natural forces of industry evolution. While the frequency of mergers and acquisitions has increased, the traditional physician role in private practice drives cottage industry principles of organization that continue to determine the lion's share of resource decisions. The interplay between cottage and corporate industrial dynamics poses an enormous complication for business strategy in the medical marketplace. That complication forms the backdrop for this book.

If we were to periodize American medicine in the post-war era, the Reagan Administration marks a significant dividing line. Prior to 1980, "regulation" shaped industry performance. While business activity was certainly prominent, strategy could take a lot for granted because the pie was growing and the marketplace accommodated the strong and not-so-strong alike. After 1980, public policy shifted. Notwithstanding the influence of regulations, laws, and licensure, emphasis in both federal policy and industry behavior switched to "competition," meaning that the path to healthcare reform would be through the marketplace. The importance of business strategy grew immeasurably in this changed industry context. Before 1980, you could be wrong strategically and still win. From, say, 1990, though, being wrong has been likely to prove more and more costly. The challenge now facing business strategy in American medicine is not only to be more right than wrong, but to be right given the particular industry dynamics of healthcare.

Looking backward, business strategy did not have any deep resonance in American medicine until the 1980s. The typical channel for strategy was "planning," but planning in the healthcare industry evolved through a series of stages, strategic planning being a relative latecomer. Figure I–1 represents in broad outline the evolution of planning stages since 1900, with each stage adding to, not replacing, the one before.

It is no accident that strategic planning first began to take hold in healthcare during the early 1980s. The rules changed then, as did the expectations healthcare providers and other industry players had of themselves in the marketplace. HMO and PPO growth, hospital mergers and acquisitions, various industry alliances, and a general belief in entrepreneurialism all helped to define a new business orientation with strategic concerns at its core. This contrasted with "healthcare planning," which had an ostensible public health orientation and included elements of area-wide and institutional planning at its core. Figure I–2 describes the transition to this new outlook.

Figure I–1.   Healthcare Industry Planning Stages

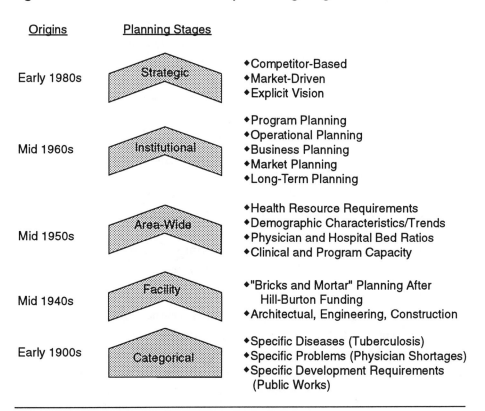

Origins	Planning Stages	
Early 1980s	Strategic	◆Competitor-Based ◆Market-Driven ◆Explicit Vision
Mid 1960s	Institutional	◆Program Planning ◆Operational Planning ◆Business Planning ◆Market Planning ◆Long-Term Planning
Mid 1950s	Area-Wide	◆Health Resource Requirements ◆Demographic Characteristics/Trends ◆Physician and Hospital Bed Ratios ◆Clinical and Program Capacity
Mid 1940s	Facility	◆"Bricks and Mortar" Planning After Hill-Burton Funding ◆Architectual, Engineering, Construction
Early 1900s	Categorical	◆Specific Diseases (Tuberculosis) ◆Specific Problems (Physician Shortages) ◆Specific Development Requirements (Public Works)

Figure I–2.   Transition from Healthcare Planning to
                    Strategic Planning

"Healthcare Planning"   ⟶   "Strategic Planning"

◆Public Health Orientation ⟶ ◆Business Orientation
◆Area Needs ⟶ ◆Demand
◆Morbidity/Mortality Trends ⟶ ◆Market Segments
◆Program Development ⟶ ◆Product Line Management
◆Community Groups ⟶ ◆Customers

Three points should be emphasized about the transition to strategic planning. First, the techniques and methods of earlier planning approaches were by no means rendered obsolete. In strategic planning, for example, demand forecasts, environmental or market analyses, and alternative scenarios all depend on aspects of "healthcare planning." What changed was the frame of reference, namely, a much more explicit business orientation. Second, as the term implies, with strategic planning the focal point becomes the *idea* of strategy. Strategy is not something you can touch like a facility, an institution, or a program. It exists in the mind, but insofar as an organization's objective in planning is the formulation of strategy, strategic ideas take on a material quality that did not exist before. Finally, the single greatest factor stimulating the spread of strategic planning in healthcare was the growth of HMOs and PPOs. Referred to in the early 1980s as "alternative delivery systems," these managed care arrangements altered the marketplace to such an extent that hospitals, health insurance companies, and eventually physicians realized they, too, like businesses in other industries, had to think strategically.

Given that managed care influences so much of the business of medicine, the term, plus the trend toward managed care, require a few comments of their own. The term itself is a product of the 1980s where pressures to achieve cost containment came from both the healthcare industry and the Washington policy establishment. Indeed, concerns for cost containment, the change from regulation to competition in national policy, and the emergence of managed care all were part of a single development. One difficulty with the term "managed care," however, is that it is used in a variety of ways.[1]

---

[1] For a classic discussion of managed care, see Alain C. Enthoven, *Theory and Practice of Managed Competition in Healthcare* (Amsterdam and New York: Science Publishing Co., 1988). For a broad cross section of healthcare industry perspectives on managed care, see an edited volume by Peter Boland, *Making Managed Healthcare Work* (Gaithersburg, Maryland: Aspen Publishers, 1993). Two comprehensive bibliographies on managed care are included in David E. Vogel, *Family Physicians and Managed Care* (Kansas City: The American Academy of Family Physicians, 1993); and *An Inconsistent Picture: A Compilation of Analyses of Economic Impacts of Competing Approaches to Healthcare Reform By Experts and Stakeholders* (Office of Technology Assessment/Government Printing Office, 1993).

I would argue that the term itself has a double meaning. On the one hand, it refers to any number of specific *organizational or economic initiatives adopted to bring about cost containment* in the delivery of healthcare services. In that sense managed care includes, but is certainly not limited to: 1) HMOs and PPOs; 2) DRG, discount fee-for-service and capitation reimbursement; 3) benefit incentives to migrate hospital services from inpatient to outpatient or from hospital to ambulatory settings; 4) various forms of utilization review including pre-authorization, concurrent review, retrospective review, and catastrophic case management; 5) specialty provider discount arrangements ranging from mental health services to tertiary transplant procedures; and 6) "gatekeeper" arrangements in which a primary care physician (PCP) has the responsibility for coordinating all medical services individuals receive.

On the other hand, managed care refers to a *phase in healthcare industry evolution* beyond solo practice, fee-for-service medicine. Use of the term managed care in this way is not unlike the way historians make reference to the "industrial age" or "progressive era." American medicine then, is now in the age of managed care.

Two other managed care terms discussed in this book should be mentioned as well: "managed care systems" and "managed competition."

❏ Managed care systems are *types of delivery systems* incorporating at the very least one element of managed care. HMOs, PPOs, point-of-service (POS) plans, and EPOs (exclusive provider organizations) are the obvious examples. But traditional indemnity health insurance coupled with preauthorization provisions also qualifies as a managed care system. As industry evolution under managed care reaches maturity, it is conceivable that for those who live and work in the United States, upwards of 90 percent of healthcare services will be realized through one or another type of managed care system.

❏ Managed competition is the expression of *health policy* now in favor not only at the federal level, but in a growing number of states that have passed their own managed competition legislation. The policy of managed competition is designed to stimulate enrollment—public and private sector employees, Medicaid, and even Medicare—into approved managed care systems. The assumption behind this policy is that with individuals obtaining care through managed care systems, those systems will compete for enrollees, creating efficiencies and savings that will lower prices and improve the quality of service provided.

The relationship between managed care, managed care systems, and managed competition is depicted in Figure I–3.

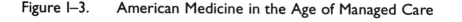

Figure I–3.   American Medicine in the Age of Managed Care

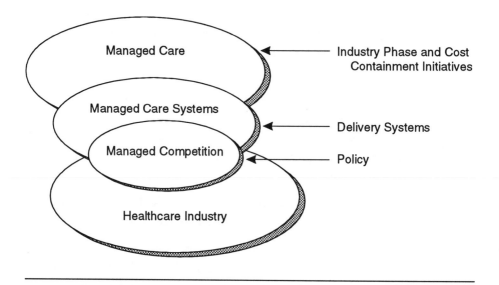

While national policies can be expected to continue stimulating the growth of managed care, it should be kept in mind that managed care is an *industry* activity. Business strategy was not a prominent feature of healthcare planning prior to managed care industry activity, but its role has escalated with the increased influence of such activity. The more healthcare industry evolution progresses under the aegis of managed care, the more important strategic thinking and business strategy in American medicine becomes.

This book is for anyone working in the healthcare industry whose work involves strategic thinking, or who might in the course of their work need to develop a business strategy. Most of the text is written from the standpoint of hospitals, physicians, and health insurance companies, though its themes also apply to pharmaceutical companies and various ancillary service providers. The book consists of six chapters, with each chapter designed to accomplish two things: 1) summarize the message and major elements of an author or coauthor's writing on a key aspect of strategic thinking in business; and 2) apply the summaries on business strategy to critical discussions bearing on business strategy in American medicine. These discussions represent the major part of the book.

The authors selected—1) Benjamin Tregoe and John Zimmerman; 2) Kenichi Ohmae; 3) Al Ries and Jack Trout; 4) Bruce Henderson; 5) Michael Porter; and 6) Stan Davis and Bill Davidson—have each in some way left their mark on the field of business strategy as a whole. They are big thinkers whose work I believe can contribute significantly to strategic thinking in the healthcare industry. Every effort has been made to preserve the scope and texture of their work. The chapter-by-chapter summaries serve as platforms for addressing various strategic concerns relating to business in healthcare. The healthcare discussions build on one another, progressing from essential qualities in strategic thinking to my argument for post-industrial strategic thinking under managed care.

No doubt other authors could have been chosen. The six who were selected, though, were chosen because their work is preeminently strategic in nature, and because the authors collectively lent themselves to the themes I wanted to develop—themes that speak directly to the difficult challenges business strategy confronts in the medical marketplace today.

One last point: Strategic thinking exists not just in strategic planning but in market planning and business planning as well. While there are basic differences between each of the "big three" types of planning, there should not be any difference in the quality of strategic thinking that informs each. As I see it, strategic thinking is best if approached on its own terms and then allowed to drive the content of a strategic plan, no less than a market plan or a business plan. When the process of strategy formulation is reversed, more times than not the quality of strategic thinking in all planning—strategic, market, and business—suffers. This book, therefore, should be a useful tool for those engaged in all such planning endeavors. Figure I–4 and the discussion in Appendix A, illustrate the book's focus on strategic thinking and business strategy.

Figure 1–4.   Strategic Thinking and Its Relationship to
Strategic, Market, and Business Planning

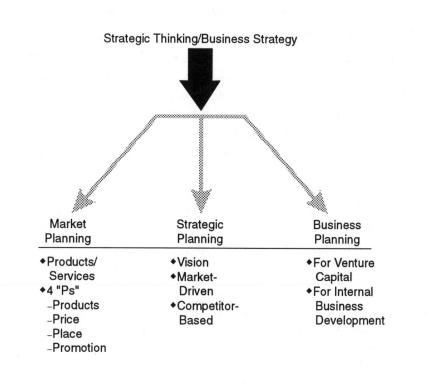

Strategic Thinking/Business Strategy

Market Planning	Strategic Planning	Business Planning
◆Products/ Services ◆4 "Ps" –Products –Price –Place –Promotion	◆Vision ◆Market- Driven ◆Competitor- Based	◆For Venture Capital ◆For Internal Business Development

CHAPTER 1

The Concept of Strategy

The U.S. healthcare system includes an enormous diversity of organizations. Many are businesses with profit as their basic concern. Others are not-for-profit, but with no less of a business orientation. Still others are government institutions operating within such severe budgetary constraints it could be argued they confront the harshest bottom line of all. Some healthcare organizations produce services. Others produce commodities. In addition, there are many different payors, providers, and vendors selling products and services to payors, providers, and patients.

Pluralism is a fact of life in the U.S. healthcare system. Often it is used ideologically to celebrate the system's diversity. Other times it is used descriptively to emphasize the system's complexity. Still other times it is used analytically to highlight the system's evolution toward new institutional relationships. Ideally, pluralism should mean not only that there are countless business organizations in the marketplace pursuing their own specific strategies, but that these strategies have all been individually crafted to link specific strengths to desired ends.

Benjamin Tregoe, John Zimmerman, and their colleagues focus on this last point.[1] In developing their message, they emphasize two themes: 1) the difference between *strategic* thinking and *operational* thinking; and 2) the role of the *driving force* in strategy formulation. Insofar as these themes are neglected by those who make the key decisions in the medical marketplace, the much-vaunted pluralism of American medicine is likely to produce a hodgepodge of strategies that diminish not only the performance of individual businesses, but the system as a whole.

WHAT VERSUS HOW

There are many definitions of strategy:

- ❏ "A strategy is a unified, comprehensive, and integrated plan relating the strategic advantages of the firm to the challenges of its environment. It is designed to ensure that the basic objectives of the enterprise are achieved."[2]

- ❏ "An organization's strategy is a statement of the fundamental means it will use, subject to a set of environmental constraints, to try to achieve its objectives. Alternatively, an organization's strategy is the fundamental pattern of present and planned resource deployments and environmental interactions that indicates how the organization will achieve its objectives."[3]

---

[1] Benjamin B. Tregoe and John W. Zimmerman. *Top Management Strategy: What It Is and How to Make It Work* (New York: Simon and Schuster, 1980); and Benjamin B. Tregoe, John W. Zimmerman, Ronald A. Smith and Peter M. Tobia. *Vision in Action: How to Integrate Your Company's Strategic Goals into Day-to-Day Management Decisions* (New York: Simon & Schuster, 1989). For simplicity sake, when I refer to *Vision in Action* I will limit my reference to Tregoe and Zimmerman.

[2] William F. Glueck. *Strategic Management and Business Policy*. Cited in James B. Webber and Joseph P. Peters. *Strategic Thinking: New Frontier for Hospital Management* (Chicago: American Hospital Publishing, 1983), 9.

[3] Charles Hofer and Dan Schendel. *Strategy Formulation: Analytic Concepts*. Cited in Webber and Peters, et al., 1983: 9.

❏ "Providing direction is the traditional objective assigned to corporate strategy: To give the company a sense of purpose and mission. Providing cohesion, on the other hand, is an objective of corporate strategy which is often ignored. Yet, it is not only important but also more essential than providing direction."[4]

❏ "(S)trategy is the pattern of major objectives, purposes, or goals and essential policies and plans for achieving those goals."[5]

❏ "(F)or our purposes, strategy-making is a response that does not necessarily 'solve' the problem, but which redefines it in terms of more familiar subproblems. Unlike rational-analytic problem solving, the function of strategy is not to 'solve' a problem, but to so structure a situation that the emergent problems are solvable."[6]

Whatever the merit of these statements, I believe they are inadequate—not so much because they define strategy in language more akin to government proposals or academic social science than business, but because they blur the distinction between strategy and organization.

To their credit, Tregoe and Zimmerman take the concept of strategy out of an organizational context and give it a context of its own. Strategy refers to "what" an organization wants to be, not "how" it conducts itself in getting there. The what/how distinction is central to their argument that too many organizations allow the details of the operating environment to overwhelm strategy. While strategy and operational issues are obviously related, Tregoe and Zimmerman emphasize that strategy alone should set the direction for business organizations:

> Strategy should provide a picture of the organization as it wants to look in the future. Strategy is vision directed at *what* the organization should be, and not *how* the organization will get there. We define strategy as the framework which guides those choices that determine the nature and direction of an organization (1980, 17).

---

4 Hugo Uyterhoeven et al. *Strategy and Organization: Text and Cases in General Management.* Cited in Webber and Peters, 1983: 9.

5 Kenneth R. Andrews. *The Concept of Corporate Strategy.* Cited in Webber and Peters, 1983: 8.

6 Richard P. Rummelt. *Strategic Management: A New View of Business Policy and Planning.* Cited in Webber and Peters, 1983: 16.

Since the publication of their first book in 1980, changes in the philosophy of American management, particularly the acceptance of more participatory Japanese approaches, make it useful to clarify one point. It is possible to read into Tregoe and Zimmerman's thinking a rigid hierarchical view of management in which those at the top set strategy, and those at the bottom follow. That is not their intent at all. The process of formulating strategy, they suggest, can and should involve input from individuals at all levels. Indeed, they emphasize this participatory theme in their second book, *Vision in Action*.

Notwithstanding the importance of employee participation, Tregoe and Zimmerman's point is that strategy formulation too often becomes entangled in day-to-day business operations. To the extent that the strategy/operations distinction breaks down: 1) senior managers become less oriented to thinking strategically; 2) current objectives define future direction, rather than future direction defining current objectives; and 3) the vision behind a business gets lost, reducing strategy to the justification of budgets and resource allocations.

Perhaps the authors' most compelling comment involves the tendency of organizations to adapt strategy to routine business difficulties. These "operational fixes," they warn, are dangerous because, "If an organization is headed in the wrong direction, the last thing it needs is to get there more efficiently" (1980, 19).

WHAT VERSUS HOW IN HEALTHCARE

The what-versus-how distinction is especially relevant to the healthcare industry. Walk into any hospital and speak to middle and senior level management—all the talk you will hear is about "putting out fires." Suggest special cost-saving provider arrangements to employers, and most VPs of human resources will decline because their "plate is full right now." Propose innovations to health insurers requiring that they rethink their traditional functions of claims processing and provider relations, and the response is that "it conflicts with what the organization is presently doing." The pattern is evident throughout the healthcare system. Whether due to reimbursement cuts or rising costs, changes in technology or developments in managed care, local competition or older plant and equipment, strategy is increasingly subordinated to operational difficulties in day-to-day business.

Two examples from my own consulting experiences illustrate this tendency. The first involves a major academic medical center located in a very competitive market. This medical center, as is often the case with such institutions, has a very high cost structure that turned-off local payors. We were retained by one of the academic departments of the medical staff (an extremely prestigious department) to obtain "center of excellence arrangements" with these same local payors: HMOs, PPOs, union trust funds, and others. Our goal was for payors to channel their more difficult, tertiary cases to the highly skilled subspecialists comprising the department's faculty. Our argument to the payors was that most physicians in HMOs and PPOs are generalists in their chosen specialty and not the best people to treat unusual or tertiary conditions. A center of excellence arrangement would provide the means for referring such cases, reducing complication rates, and improving patients' overall quality of care.

Part of our responsibility was to formulate a discount that included professional and facility components. The physicians were willing to discount their professional charges because they recognized this would be the only way to ensure channeling. The medical center, on the other hand, was resistant to discounting facility charges. Management cited three reasons: 1) it did not fully understand operating room costs and was therefore uncomfortable providing additional discounts because costs for the same procedure varied from case to case; 2) it could not commit to significant discounts until there was a guarantee that some percentage of new cases would be generated; and 3) it did not want to jeopardize established HMO/PPO relationships with discounts that went beyond existing agreements.

Preoccupied with an operations mindset, management could not accept the limitations inherent in its reasoning: 1) costs for the same surgical procedure naturally vary from case to case; 2) the amount of new volume resulting from these special arrangements can never be guaranteed; and 3) lower prices are just about the only way, in a competitive environment, to capture increased market share. It bears emphasizing that the medical center was substantially under capacity, so even significantly discounted facility charges would have been better than the dust the facility was collecting.

Eventually, we were forced to obtain "professional only" agreements in which the physicians discounted their services, but the hospital did not. Since the facility charge is such a large proportion of the total cost of tertiary cases, the rationale for channeling was diluted. In this one market, then, HMO and PPO members who could have benefited from having access to university-based subspecialists, now have limited access at best.

A second example of strategy getting entangled in operations involves the health insurance industry. It is generally recognized that the rise in administrative costs associated with health insurance is one source of healthcare inflation. While different constituencies will debate the trends in administrative expenses, the insurance industry recognizes that its administrative costs are a problem. However, rather than viewing the problem strategically and then allowing an operational approach to evolve, the industry has viewed the problem operationally, forcing strategy to follow.

A variety of initiatives have been undertaken over the past 10 years by both commercial carriers and Blue Cross Blue Shield plans to automate the industry's traditionally labor-intensive claims processing operation. These efforts, known as "electronic claims processing," have focused on existing functions such as confirming patients' eligibility, routing claims from providers to insurers, ensuring that "clean" claims are submitted, and paying claims electronically. Despite electronic claims processing simplifying and even reducing the variable costs of this operation, it has not slowed down the cost escalation in administration overall.

Two related issues are involved here. The first involves the insurance industry's frame of reference in determining how automation should be applied to claims processing. Picture, for a moment, Henry Ford and his prototype Model T. Ford wants to "manufacture" this new automobile. He bases his approach, though, on the craft model he was raised on in and around the agrarian communities of Detroit in the late nineteenth century. He solicits individual craftsmen who specialize in making carriages for the horse and buggy. He trains these craftsmen on the design of the Model T. He trains them on the use of all the equipment needed to produce the Model T. He then distributes this equipment to the carriage shops he has contracted with, assured that teams of four or five will work diligently on manufacturing his automobile. Finally, he makes arrangements to sell handcrafted Model Ts in the largest horse and buggy showrooms of Detroit.

Obviously, there is something wrong here. Ford did not use a craft model of manufacturing. Instead, he redefined his operation by developing mass production capabilities and then, through vertical integration, extended the total operation backward to obtain raw materials cheaply and forward to stimulate mass marketing. For Ford, *strategy preceded operations.* Imagine what would have happened if the then prevailing operational model dictated his strategy. Yet, that is just what occurs today with the health insurance industry's approach to electronic claims processing—only now, the assembly-line logic of paper claims processing dictates the strategy for automation.

This leads to a second issue: The insurance industry's vision in determining which goals automation should support. Businesses have choices. They can be organizational introverts, limiting vision to parts of the whole, or they can be organizational extroverts, extending vision to relationships between the parts. Introverts confine change to existing relationships; extroverts change relationships. It is my belief, at least insofar as claims processing is concerned, that most players in the health insurance industry are introverts. Rather than the industry extending automation to claims processing as part of restructuring the total information system, the industry has confined automation to the claims process itself.

While there may be exceptions, the health insurance industry's goal in electronic claims processing has not been to make a qualitative break with existing operations. The goal has been to automate what is essentially the industry's back-office function. Consequently, a whole series of possibilities involving automated payment and reporting systems have not been pursued. It is possible, for instance, to combine electronic claim processing with a credit card to deliver on-line, real time transaction capability at the point of service. This would allow patient eligibility, coverage determination, preauthorization of procedures and authorization of payment to all occur before patients leave their doctor's office. Claim adjudication, logging explanation of benefits in a patient's credit card account, and remittance to providers could all occur within five days of the patient visit. Patients would not have to go through the cumbersome process of submitting claims and reconciling what their insurance pays with what they had to lay out. Nor would they have any out-of-pocket costs for one month. Employers would have greater flexibility in offering health benefit plans. Physicians could be paid within a week of the patient encounter, eliminating their accounts-receivable problem. And utilization reporting, linking initial and subsequent patient encounters, could track physician performance at the process level where many consider the truest measure of quality to be. In short, the entire payment process could be vastly simplified for all parties concerned, yielding more powerful synergies in overall information management. Such a change, however, requires changing basic functional relationships—something the operational side of the industry believes is too difficult to do.

Tregoe and Zimmerman suggest that one of the dangers of operational thinking is its "rearview-mirror" quality. As you move ahead but base strategic decisions on current operations, you are assuming things will continue as they have in the past. In healthcare, nothing could be further from the truth.

STRATEGY VERSUS ROUTINIZATION

The most important theme Tregoe and Zimmerman develop in their two books is that senior management should not confuse strategic with operational thinking. When that happens, operational thinking infuses itself in strategy, eventually defining it. The result is what might be called the "routinization of strategy." Routinization is not the same as implementation or institutionalization. These occur *after* strategy has been formulated. The routinization of strategy occurs *before* implementation or institutionalization, when a business's strategy is being formulated. With the routinization of strategy, the organization or bureaucracy of a business takes over for the ideas that should set the pace for that business.

The great German sociologist Max Weber warned that routinization is an underlying trend of modern society.[7] He viewed routinization as possibly modern society's gravest threat because it suffocates the role of ideas, leadership, and independent judgment. As routinization progresses, Weber argued, there is nothing to counterbalance the power that bureaucracies acquire over people. He likened this trend to an "iron cage" in which a mechanical, formal rationality gains hegemony over all aspects of public and private life, government, and commerce.

When strategy is routinized, management creates its own iron cage. Rather than strategy helping management direct the organization of a business, strategy provides the intellectual justification for the organization to take on

---

7 Max Weber. *From Max Weber: Essays in Sociology.* H.H. Ferth and W. Wright Mills, eds. (New York: Oxford University Press, 1946).

a life of its own. With the routinization of strategy 1) management is prevented from entertaining new and different business opportunities, 2) variations of the same old operational logic dictate future business direction, and 3) the organization as a whole suffers from a lack of long-term vision. The routinization strategy is the path toward mediocrity in business, and it is to Tregoe and Zimmerman's credit that they tried to block that path. Having said that, I would push this theme further than the authors themselves take it.

Despite the importance of the strategy/operations distinction, Tregoe and Zimmerman never accounted for why the line between strategic and operational thinking gets blurred. In their first book, *Top Management Strategy*, they suggest that the culprit is "long-range planning." During the course of this process, operational problems and biases frame how strategic issues are considered. In effect, they attribute the diminution of strategy in business organizations to the process through which planning occurs. While they make a number of very cogent remarks about the effects of long-range planning on strategy, they do not explain why strategic thinking is so easily co-opted by operational thinking in the planning process.

Conventional wisdom, which I think Tregoe and Zimmerman would agree with, focuses on a variety of organizational factors: businesses function on the basis of conservative decision rules; organizations in general are shaped by the politics of narrow institutional interests; business organizations tend to be reactive; business organizations, like biological organisms, shy away from the uncertain; and business organizations tend to be short-term oriented, preoccupied with the next quarter's results, not the next decade's prospects.

The problem I have with this reasoning is its inevitability. It suggests that by virtue of strategy functioning in organizations, it naturally becomes routinized. Instead, I would argue that strategy becomes routinized when management allows the *boundary* between strategy and organization to collapse. When that collapse occurs, strategic thinking merges with operational thinking; organizational dynamics then come into play and strategy becomes routinized—but not until that occurs.

On the other hand, when the boundary between strategy and organization is maintained, there is a tangible difference between the two. Strategy stands apart from the organization and has a *structural* relationship to it. This structural relationship enlarges the concept of strategy to include not only the picture of the organization as management wants it to look in the future—its vision, or the "what" Tregoe and Zimmerman refer to—but also the core ideas management needs to *critique* the organization.

By critique, I mean management asking big-picture type questions about the nature and direction of the business and asking them on the basis of independent critical judgment. What assumptions were made by management to commit to the present course, and how have circumstances affected those assumptions? If we stay on track, will we get to where we want to be? What changes should we adopt in our organization or operations to stay on track? Should we change our course; and if we do, what changes in both organization and operations are required? What core issues confront the business, and what changes in the organization are needed to effectively deal with these issues? What are the key values and goals of the organization? What were they? What should they be? How is the organization's performance conforming to those values and goals, and how should performance change to better meet them?

When strategy is used by management for both critique and long-term vision, management takes control of the business rather than the deadly weight of the organization taking control of it. Renewal, not routinization, becomes the order of the day.

A shortcoming in Tregoe and Zimmerman is that while they addressed the strategy/operations distinction from the standpoint of vision, they neglected it from the standpoint of critique. I would add three points, then, to the concept of strategy they layed out. These are depicted in Figure 1–1.

- ❑ First, strategy is a necessary counterpoint to the organization of any business. Strategy's role is to serve management as an ongoing source of critique for the organization and to provide long-term vision for the business.

- ❑ Second, it is management's responsibility to maintain the boundary between strategy and organization since the ideas on one side of the boundary are every bit as real as operations on the other side. Business deteriorates—any business, whether it be IBM or the corner grocery store—when management allows the boundary between strategy and organization to collapse.

Figure 1–1.   Boundary between Strategy and Organization

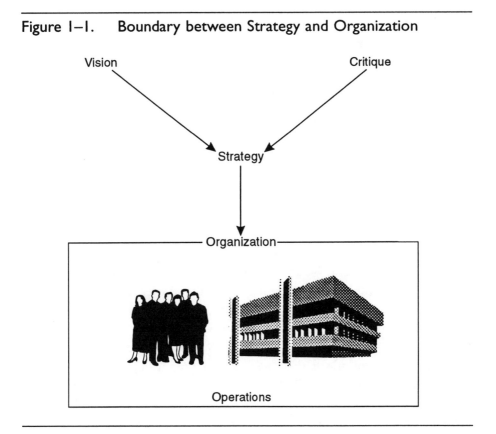

□ Finally, and here I am going beyond the framework Tregoe and Zimmerman layed out, the strategy/operations distinction does not mean that operational thinking should be categorically excluded from strategic thinking.[8] What it means is that it should help to inform strategic thinking, *but on the strategy side of the boundary*. From this vantage point, operational thinking has the capacity to enrich and toughen the overall quality of strategy. Conversely, if a business has no real boundary between strategy and its organization, operational input into strategic thinking will inevitably lead to the routinization of strategy and to a decline in the business as a whole.

---

8 Recall that Tregoe and Zimmerman do not view strategic thinking as a rigid, top-down management exercise, but believe it should include individuals and input from all levels of the organization.

STRATEGY VERSUS ROUTINIZATION
IN HEALTHCARE

Tregoe and Zimmerman have argued that the subordination of strategy to operations is a constant threat to business. In the last section, I suggested that this subordination occurs when the boundary between strategy and organization is not maintained. When that happens, strategic thinking gets bogged down in the details of day-to-day operations, and the routinization of strategy sets in. It is the routinization of strategy that underlies long-term business decline. This process has its own particular logic in the healthcare system.

One of the enduring features of the current industry structure in healthcare is that it is part cottage industry and part corporate, and that it is the cottage part—physicians—that continues to drive the corporate part—insurance companies, hospitals, hospital systems, and even Fortune 500 pharmaceutical companies. However, physicians are not particularly interested in strategic thinking. While there will always be exceptions, when most physicians think strategically the one issue they focus on is reimbursement and how reimbursement affects their medical practice. A key factor behind the routinization of strategy in healthcare, therefore, is the institutional space that strategy occupies. Physicians, who represent the industry's "independent variable," are not especially interested in strategic thinking; while insurers, hospital systems, and others in the corporate sector, the industry's "dependent variable," are clearly interested. In the first instance, strategy becomes routinized through lack of resolve, in the second instance, through lack of fit.

Consistent with its industry structure, the organizational context in healthcare provides additional impetus for the routinization of strategy. If a potentially valuable body of knowledge is to form the basis of a business, it must literally be institutionalized by that business. Once such knowledge is inside the organization, strategy can then shape operations to produce products and services as well as sales in the market. No matter how potentially valuable the knowledge, though, it has to be taken over and integrated within a business organization before strategy can function.[9]

---

[9] The evaluation of business plans by corporate decision makers and venture capitalists is a good case in point. A key consideration in the evaluation of any business plan is how well the proposed business organization will be able to shape potentially profitable

Healthcare is unique among all the industries I am aware of, in that its body of knowledge—medicine—resists being taken over. Unlike other industries where the knowledge domain fits inside the organizational domain, *in the healthcare industry medicine is at best only partially integrated.* This partial integration I attribute to three factors: 1) medicine's technological imperative; 2) medicine's professional interests conflicting with those of business; and 3) medicine's special role in society. All three factors represent some of the grand themes in the history of American medicine. From a business standpoint, they are significant because they all contribute to the routinization of strategy in healthcare.

Medicine's Technological Imperative

There has always been a tension between the "art" and the "science" in medicine. This tension has its origins in an imperative presupposed in science to control nature and, in the case of medical science, to cure illness and disease. In recent years, that tension has given way to the art being subordinated to the science because of the extraordinary clinical power medical technology brings to patient care.

For their part, doctors want the latest and best technology; hospitals, if they are to survive, have to offer it; and patients expect it. While it may well be that the more technologically sophisticated medicine becomes, the more effective it becomes, what the *hubris* of medical technology means for business strategy is that technological opportunities and threats define the terms through which strategy is formulated. On the provider side, strategy tends to focus on purchasing this or that new high-tech instrument; obtaining maximum reimbursement from payors; and substituting newer, more sophisticated procedures for older ones. On the payor side, strategy tends to focus on limiting the diffusion of new and expensive technologies, using lower-cost substitute technologies, and shifting patients from the more expensive procedural side of healthcare to the less expensive medical side.

In this context, the routinization of strategy in healthcare occurs because the *boundary between strategy and technology has not been adequately maintained.*

---

knowledge. If such knowledge cannot be completely shaped by the business so that it supports the business strategy, capital will not be forthcoming, and the business will not be funded.

Rather than strategy functioning as an independent source of vision and critique that shapes the direction of medical technology, strategy is too often driven by the details technology sets forth. The result is that strategy functions as ideology, reinforcing medicine's technological imperative. Insofar as spiraling healthcare costs and other system problems in the United States continue to have an "out-of-control" quality, at least part of the explanation rests with medicine's technological imperative and its influence on the routinization of strategy.

Professional versus Business Interests

Medicine as a profession and as a business represents two entirely different systems. The profession revolves around physicians who expect to serve patients as free and independent practitioners on a fee-for-service basis. The business revolves around diverse corporate organizations that impose a division of labor around and through physicians' professional role. The two systems are also governed by different principles of organization:

Profession	Business
Autonomy	Hierarchy
Self-regulation	Competition
Internal norms	Commercial values
Technical considerations	Bottom-line objectives

These different principles do not mean that the business has a profit orientation but the profession does not. They mean that the two pursue profit differently. Where the medical profession is unwilling to transform physicians' autonomous craft role into more narrowly circumscribed hierarchical roles in larger corporate institutions, business interests look to do so at every turn. If we think in terms of "the container" and "the thing contained," medicine is only partly in the business container because the economic interests of the medical profession and business conflict.[10]

For both the medical profession and business, therefore, what might be characterized as dysfunctional politics gets in the way of strategic thinking.

---

[10]Notable exceptions would be the pharmaceutical and biotechnology industries.

Here, the routinization of strategy in healthcare occurs because the *boundary between strategy and politics has not been adequately maintained.* Rather than strategy providing an independent source of vision and critique that shapes the direction of medicine in business, strategy gets entangled in political variables emanating from the conflict between medicine and business. To the extent that this conflict continues, strategic thinking in the healthcare industry will continue to be routinized, and business will be prevented from taking medicine to a more advanced level.

Medicine's Special Role in Society

The third factor behind medicine's partial integration into business involves its special role in society. The notion of an industry having a "special role" is not unique. The military has a special role, so does agriculture. In each case, government and the marketplace coalesce to exempt industry performance from Adam Smith's invisible hand. For different reasons, medicine's special role in society exempts the healthcare industry as well.

This special role can be traced to at least three sources. First, patients do not turn to medical businesses when they have a medical problem; they turn to medicine. Second, federal and state governments do not delegate the responsibility for professional licensure and certification to medical businesses; they delegate it to the medical profession. Finally, if there was ever an industry in which the proverbial cart was put before the horse, it is the healthcare industry, in that medicine has typically led the way and business has typically followed. To cite but two examples: the modern hospital developed not as a business, but as "the physicians' workshop"; and health insurance developed, not because it is profitable, but because health services had to be made affordable. In both cases, medicine was the catalyst for change, and business got involved after the fact.

From this standpoint, the routinization of strategy in healthcare can be attributed to medicine's special role in society. Instead of strategy providing an independent source of vision and critique that shapes the direction of medicine, strategy too often depends on developments emanating from inside medicine itself. As a result, the routinization of strategy in healthcare occurs because the *boundary between strategy and medicine has not been maintained.* One of the great challenges the healthcare industry faces is for strategic thinking to accept medicine's special role and to guide the business of medicine accordingly.

THE DRIVING FORCE

Throughout this chapter, I have focused on Tregoe and Zimmerman's distinction between strategic and operational thinking and their insistence that the latter should not condition the former. When operational thinking crosses the boundary into strategy, strategy becomes routinized. With the routinization of strategy, management loses its ability to maintain a long-term vision and exercise an independent source of critique. The result is that business strategy deteriorates. Tregoe and Zimmerman's concept of the "driving force" builds on this reasoning and represents their other important contribution to the field.

The driving force helps define the nature and direction of a business, or the "what" a business wants to be. It is, in Tregoe and Zimmerman's words, the "central hook" or "essential building block" for formulating strategy. To understand the term "driving force" it should be kept in mind that the essence of any business is the products and services it offers and the markets and customers it serves. The concept of a driving force keeps management focused on that fact. The driving force is "the primary determiner of the scope of future products and markets" (1980, 40). It "provides a broad definition for future product and market direction" (1989, 40). This broad definition constitutes the common characteristics or standards management can use when deciding which product and market choices are consistent with the vision of a business and which are not. With the driving force clearly understood throughout the organization, everyone in the business speaks a common strategic language.

Tregoe and Zimmerman identify seven *potential* driving forces. These driving forces represent underlying strategic areas for any business. They fall into three categories:[11]

---

[11]Tregoe and Zimmerman, 1980, 43; and Tregoe and Zimmerman, 1989, 209–214. In their most recent formulation, the authors actually refer to eight driving forces. I have omitted any reference to "natural resources" as a driving force, however, because it has no relevance to strategic and business issues in healthcare.

Category	Strategic Area/Driving Force
Products/Markets	Products-offered
	Markets-served
Capabilities	Technology
	Low-cost production capability
	Operations capability
	Method of sale/distribution
Results	Return/profit

While all seven driving forces could be central to any business, the authors emphasize that an organization should rely on "*one and only one driving force at any given time*" (1980, 43). This does not mean that there is only one possible driving force for a business, or even that there is only one correct driving force. It means that management should commit to having only one driving force, and that switching from one to another is problematic. In effect, a business's driving force is management's wager on the future. It should not make multiple wagers, nor should it switch wagers. Inconsistency on either count causes confusion and pushes in conflicting directions. Which driving force should a business select? The one which takes greatest advantage of a business's strengths as opposed to its weaknesses, and which best exploits industry opportunities while avoiding industry threats. Making that determination should be one of the major objectives in strategic thinking.

The seven driving forces are described below:[12]

- ❑ **Products-offered.** A products-offered driving force seeks new markets, market segments, and customer groups for existing products. Such products have a quality or uniqueness that differentiates them from competitors. Product development and innovation should seek a competitive edge and strive to preserve that edge. Because market expansion is a necessity under this driving force, organizations that are product driven usually have considerable marketing prowess. (Examples: Procter & Gamble; American Express; Disney; and NFL, NBA, and MLB Properties.)

---

[12]All the summaries are drawn directly from Tregoe and Zimmerman, 1980, 43–54; and Tregoe and Zimmerman, 1989, 209–214. Some of the examples included in the summaries are Tregoe and Zimmerman's, and some are my own.

- **Markets-served.** A markets-served driving force seeks new and different products to meet the needs of a business's existing market. Businesses governed by this driving force have unusually strong ties to the market they already serve. Market research and product development focus first on helping existing customers determine their needs, and then on finding new and different products to meet those needs. With the products-offered driving force, the emphasis is on existing products and new and different markets. With the markets-served driving force, the emphasis is on existing markets and new and different products. (Examples: Citibank; the local hardware store; the American Association of Retired Persons.)

- **Technology.** Businesses with technology as their driving force capitalize on proprietary technology and on product applications from such technology. Businesses commit to this driving force because the technology they control consistently yields products or services with better-than-average sales and profit potential. Technology-driven companies need to stay at the forefront of their chosen technology. At one point, they may seek exclusive control over it. At another point, they might license it or form a joint venture around particular product applications. The upside potential for this driving force depends on the long-term business prospects of the technology. The downside threat is the risk of customers switching, product substitution, or technological obsolescence. (Examples: 3M Corporation; Microsoft; Apple Computer; and Amgen.)

- **Low-cost production capability.** This driving force reflects production capabilities that yield special cost advantages relative to competitors. Advantages include economies of scale, advanced process technologies, specific engineering approaches, unique discount arrangements, and a cost-conscious management. Usually, low-cost production is associated with high-volume, low-margin businesses where the target market is price sensitive. Businesses with this driving force can accommodate one product or many and one customer or many. The business priorities are to increase market penetration with existing or modified products or to offer current products to new markets. (Examples: McDonald's; Wal-Mart; and Charles Schwab.)

- **Operations capability.** Businesses that rely on their operations capability have some combination of human, physical, or technical strengths that set them apart in an important way. An operations capability driving force can accommodate a variety of special demands, requiring flexibility in the work process. Typically, production is customized, project oriented, and in relatively small numbers. Those with this driving force do not turn out widgets. Their products are often unique to the customer. (Examples: Bechtel; Arthur Andersen; and NASA.)

- **Method of distribution/sale.** A method of distribution/sale driving force contains strong and unique distribution or sales capabilities. Such capabilities are usually predicated on something of quality, quantity, or position inherent in the method of distribution or sale. What a business adopting this driving force commits to is that the products it sells, the customers it sells to, and the geographic boundaries of the market are all determined by the method of distribution or sale. The business is literally based on that method. (Examples: Book-of-Month-Club; Federal Express; and L.L. Bean.)

- **Return/profit.** Every business has return on investment and profit goals. Such goals, though, should not be confused with a return/profit driving force. Businesses with this driving force use return and profit considerations as their primary rationale for making product and market decisions. During the 1970s, for example, Detroit refused to produce smaller automobiles because it would mean less profit per unit. The U.S. automobile industry, in that sense, was influenced by a return/profit driving force. Typically, businesses adopting this driving force will use their resources to acquire new businesses rather than develop new products or cultivate new markets. The approach is strictly financial. (Examples: ITT; Grand Met; General Electric.)

Companies without a driving force or those with two or more driving forces or those with the wrong driving force, all fail strategically. Having failed at that level, no matter how good they are operationally, they will eventually fail in the marketplace. Once the driving force is determined, however, and assuming it is appropriate, concepts are in place for management to define the long-term vision of a business and to maintain an independent source of critique. Those concepts represent an intellectual unity that is management's responsibility to maintain. That unity is depicted in Figure 1–2.[13]

---

[13]Tregoe and Zimmerman list "five key strategic questions" in *Vision in Action*, page 38. In Figure 1–2, I have adapted their questions to the three-way relationship of driving force, vision, and critique developed in this chapter.

Figure 1–2.   Driving Force in Strategic Thinking

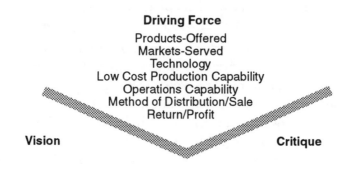

Driving Force

Products-Offered
Markets-Served
Technology
Low Cost Production Capability
Operations Capability
Method of Distribution/Sale
Return/Profit

Vision	**Critique**
1. Focus on future business.	1. Are we concentrating our resources and capabilities in a way that is most consistent with our driving force?
2. Values and norms governing strategic decisions, as well as relationships with customers and employees.	2. Do our strategic decisions, managerial approaches and customer relationships conform to our values and norms?
3. Range of acceptable current and future product/markets.	3. Do our current and future products/markets fall within the prescribed range?
4. Priorities in mix of current and future products/markets.	4. Have we adequately prioritized our current and future product/market commitments?
5. Key resources and capabilities.	5. Do we and will we have the key resources and capabilities needed to support our current and future product/market commitments?
6. Growth and return expectations.	6. Are the strategic and investment requirements inherent in the vision consistent with future growth and return expectations?

Strategy

THE DRIVING FORCE IN HEALTHCARE

The "driving force" is as relevant to strategic thinking in the healthcare industry as it is to strategic thinking in business and industry generally. With the right driving force in place, a business can focus on a single, clear direction; concentrate its strengths against an opponent's weaknesses; and leverage capabilities in a way competitors cannot. Hospitals represent a case in point.

Hospitals consume a little over 40 percent of total personal healthcare expenditures in the United States and something on the order of 5–5.5 percent of the total gross domestic product.[14] The shear size of hospital expenditures makes this industry group a constant target for further cuts. Hospitals are also complex, often unwieldy organizations with an uneven grasp of their internal costs. In addition, many hospitals have deteriorating plant and equipment, and inadequate access to capital markets. Beyond these factors, hospitals are threatened by two closely related developments:

1. Advances in medical science and technology will continue to cause hospitals to become more capital intensive and expensive. At the same time, the growth of managed care tied to capitation, all inclusive case rates, and DRG reimbursement means that hospitals will be paid proportionately less for the intensity of service they provide. Thus, the thing hospitals are expected to excel in— namely, high-tech medicine—is the very thing they are unlikely to be adequately compensated for.

2. Physicians will continue to "carve out" of the hospital setting an increasing percentage of patients they can treat on an ambulatory basis. In an environment driven by prospective reimbursement (capitation and DRGs), this represents an actuarial nightmare for hospitals because it leaves them treating mostly acute inpatients. As physician competition for the more profitable secondary hospital product increases, therefore, hospitals can expect more and more outright loses.[15]

---

[14]Suzanne Letsch, Helen Lazenby, Katherine Levit, and Cathy Cowan. "National Health Expenditures, 1991." *Healthcare Financing Review* (Winter 1992).

[15]See, for example, George Anders. "More Patients Get Quick Surgery and Go Home." *The Wall Street Journal* (August 11, 1994): B1. According to Mr. Anders, "By 1995 the AHA [American Hospital Association] predicts that outpatient surgery will rise to 75 percent of total operations."

Against that background, it has been my experience that hospital strategic thinking tends to be far too "how" oriented. Hospitals are preoccupied with myriad operational issues: reducing overhead; improving coordination among departments, establishing more advanced cost accounting and billing systems, coping with union and other labor relations issues, enhancing their physical plant, and strengthening themselves clinically. In most instances, hospital strategy is not focused on products and markets. While it is true that DRG reimbursement has prodded hospitals to manage patient stays in terms of discrete diagnostic categories, this product-line management typically pertains to hospital operations, not hospital strategy. In addition to the thicket of operational issues, the current focus of most hospital strategy is, as it has been for at least the last 50 years, on physicians and referrals.

Hospitals "market" to physicians because it is the physician who brings in patients. Ironically, the growth of a more explicit corporate bent in hospital management during the 1980s has not diminished the prominence of physician marketing in hospital strategy. Even though it has become a truism in hospital circles that "you cannot be all things to all people," trying to "be all things" through physician relationships continues to be the major thrust of most hospital strategy. Tregoe and Zimmerman's concept of the driving force can refine and improve hospitals' strategic thinking in two important respects.

First, it highlights for senior management the boundary between strategic and operational issues, pushing the latter out of the strategic and back into the operational domain. The return/profit driving force illustrates this process. As mentioned earlier, while profits and return on investment are matters every business cares about, this is not necessarily the driving force a business should be based on.

Recall the automotive industry in the mid-1970s when concern with profits per unit led Detroit to continue emphasizing larger automobiles. Return/profit, however, was not *the* driving force for any of the Big Three auto makers. Neither was products-offered, markets-served or any of the other options Tregoe and Zimmerman describe. None of the leading auto makers, in fact, committed to a single driving force to define their overall strategy. This gave the Japanese their window of opportunity to press ahead with a products-offered driving force, leading to smaller, more fuel efficient cars and substantial gains in market share. The economic losses and deteriorating market position resulting from Detroit's bollixed strategic thinking continues to haunt the U.S. economy today. In my judgment, the situation Detroit experienced in the mid-to-late-1970s is analogous to the situation hospitals face in the United States right now.

Hospitals are preoccupied with admissions and revenues. As a result, they cope with day-to-day operational problems and market to physicians, thinking this is the best way to be successful. The latest example is for hospitals to develop regional networks and to incorporate physicians into those networks through acquisition and/or PHO development.[16] If you are handicapping hospitals, though, the odds only favor this approach in the short term. In the long term, hospitals still need to define their business strategy according to the competitive demands of managed care. The lesson from Detroit is that hospitals should not focus on profits (admissions and revenues), but on winning in the managed care marketplace. Succeed that way, and profits will follow. By committing to a single driving force, hospitals avoid the preoccupations that limit strategic thinking and focus instead on what it takes to a win in the marketplace.

The second contribution of the driving force to hospitals' strategic thinking is that it forces hospitals to define themselves in terms of very specific product and market commitments. For example, in the early 1980s, Airbus, the European consortium, decided to abandon the basic 737 airplane technology Boeing had made the industry standard. Instead, it committed to a whole new generation of technology and design, which is now far superior to even the most advanced Boeing 737s. The result is that United Airlines, in a $3 billion agreement, chose Airbus to replace its entire Boeing fleet. Airbus is now the industry standard in the global market for commercial aircraft.[17]

Whether hospitals go the Airbus or Boeing route largely depends on whether they opt for a single driving force to define "what" they are. When senior management of multiple hospitals in the same community simply invest in different clinical services, they are deluding themselves in thinking

16See, for example, Elisabeth Rosenthal. "Small Hospitals Being Recruited To Join With Manhattan Giants." *New York Times* (April 4, 1994): A1.

17Jeff Cole. "Boeing's Dominance of the Aircraft Industry is Beginning to Erode. *The Wall Street Journal* (July 10, 1992): A1.

this will effectively distinguish them from competitors. Really, all they are doing is putting somewhat different bodies on the same old engine. What they should do is commit to different driving forces. Here are three illustrations:

- ❏ **Markets-served.** Let one hospital adopt a markets-served driving force. This should be the hospital with the strongest ties to the community and probably also the broadest medical staff. More than any other hospital, this hospital's strategy calls for being a truly general community hospital. It should have a diverse portfolio of clinical services, none of which are unusually capital intensive. Its president should continuously recruit the most successful internists, obstetricians, general surgeons, and others, who would serve as "low-tech" admitters. Its vice president for marketing should develop new community outreach programs (e.g., diet, stress reduction, headache/biofeedback, sports medicine, and senior healthcare). The hospital should also do everything possible to preempt the development of ambulatory surgery centers and larger, multispecialty group practices. If they do not exist, eventually the hospital may have to build them. If they do exist, the hospital might well have to acquire them. With a markets-served driving force, this general hospital has to remain a secondary hospital and resist every pressure to pursue tertiary programs. It has to blunt any competitive ambulatory care initiatives. And it has to carefully protect its standing in the community.

- ❏ **Products-offered.** Should the neighboring community hospital also adopt a markets-served driving force and compete by trying to "go one better," for example, by taking in a much respected cardiac surgery team and establishing a neonatology unit, it will eventually lose the discipline of its competitor. Clinical services will not have common cost structures; economies and efficiencies will be more difficult to achieve; needs and demands of the medical staff will become more divergent; marketing requirements will conflict; and the ability to concentrate resources will be compromised. However, if this second hospital has the capacity to adopt a products-offered driving force, other unique opportunities emerge. It could concentrate on three or four clinical areas such as cardiology, orthopedics, neurology, and oncology. Each of these areas vertically integrates and lends itself to all kinds of line extension offerings, cross-marketing relationships, and efficiencies. The hospital could then market itself as a "center of excellence." It would have considerable leverage in negotiations with HMOs and PPOs; it would be *the* hospital for patients with health problems that fall into any of the designated specialties; and, through ties to specialty groups, its geographic reach would extend well beyond the boundaries of the immediate community.

☐ **Method of distribution/sale.** Our third hospital is a medical center. It is the largest in terms of beds and the oldest in terms of physical plant. The medical center is affiliated with a major medical school 15 miles away. This affiliation provides the medical center with residents to serve its extensive Medicaid and indigent patient population. While the medical center had always been viewed as the place to go for specialty medicine, in the last 10 years the percentage of private patient admissions declined dramatically. Consequently, losses are increasing, its physical plant is deteriorating, and the hospital is in a downward spiral. The medical center clearly cannot compete based on a markets-served driving force because it does not have the relationship to the community the first hospital has. And it cannot compete based on a products-offered driving force because it is in no position to acquire or effectively promote specialty clusters like the second hospital can. But the medical center notices that both competitors have a very traditional understanding of what it means to be a hospital.

It decides to break out of that mold, out of the concept of a hospital's traditional four walls, and to adopt a method of distribution/sale driving force, meaning that it will pursue an aggressive satellite strategy. Knowing the trend towards outpatient surgery, the medical center turns to the "one-day health and hospital" concept. It uses its access to capital markets through the medical school affiliation, and co-ventures with selected physicians in the community to build two separate multispecialty group/ambulatory surgery center campuses. One campus is on each side of town. The medical center also leverages its affiliation with the medical school to promote a "university affiliates" brand identity for each of the campuses. In the medical center itself, one patient pavilion is renovated. In addition, the operating rooms are upgraded, and scheduling is improved. These latter developments help to regain physician confidence and enhance the medical center's image as a tertiary facility. The medical center is now positioned to ride the tide of long-term industry trends. It can support capitation arrangements with HMOs because of a reengineered cost structure. It can attract fee-for-service patients because of strong and predictable relationships with selected physician groups in the community. Most importantly, though, it can compete in the local market in ways competitors cannot.

The battle is now joined. How well each of these hospitals performs is not just a function of their driving force. The driving force allows management to define *what* a business is—what specific approach to products and markets the business should adopt. That is part of the wager management makes in its responsibility for business strategy. But there are other elements to that wager as well.

CHAPTER 2

The Quality of Strategy

Every industry has its own traditions that reinforce nuances specific to that industry. With PCs, for example, there is something of a renegade quality lying deep in the industry's folklore—Jobs and Wozniak developing their first Apple prototype in the garage, or Bill Gates buying a now anonymous neophyte's operating system for less than $100,000 and using it to develop MS-DOS for IBM.[1] These traditions, in turn, influence strategic thinking. IBM understood the industry's renegade quality when it freed PC development from Armonk and allowed the original product team to work independently in Boca Raton. More recently, Ben Rosen, Compaq's Chairmen, understood this same thinking when he asked two mid-level managers to scour a major industry trade show for parts and then assemble a low-cost PC in their hotel suite, resulting in Compaq eventually becoming number

---

[1] Daniel Ichbiah with Susan Knepper. *The Making of Microsoft* (Rocklin, CA: Prima Publishing, 1993), 76.

one in sales volume.[2] The contrast between the computer industry's renegade folklore and its large-scale corporate organization has frequently been the catalyst for innovative strategic thinking.

The healthcare industry presents a much different story. The "not-for-profit" tradition among community hospitals, the "property-and-casualty" tradition among insurers, and the "professional" tradition among physicians, all reinforce a kind of *nobles oblige* in the marketplace. By and large, it is only in the pharmaceutical sector where long standing traditions exist which sanction innovative strategic thinking. While recent developments involving managed care may prove to be an exception, in most instances providers and payors continue to think of themselves as having a natural franchise in the marketplace. More than anything else, I believe, this has helped to reify strategic thinking in healthcare.

It is this context that makes Kenichi Ohmae's *The Mind of the Strategist* so relevant.[3] Ohmae's great strength is that he helps the reader appreciate many of the characteristics inherent in strategic insight. Along the way, he also provides useful tools for strategy formulation. Where Tregoe and Zimmerman stake out the concept of strategy, Ohmae brings the reader *into* the qualities of strategic thinking itself.

STRATEGIC THINKING AS AN ART

Ohmae's overriding concern is to combat the intellectual stagnation he sees in much of today's strategic thinking. He attributes this stagnation to an excess of formal reasoning in strategy formulation. What is especially valuable about his argument is that it reflects the way the Japanese have approached business competition in the world markets during the last few decades. In that regard, Ohmae builds an instinctive Japanese perspective into his discussions on strategy.

For Ohmae, "analysis is the critical starting point" (11). In strategic thinking, management is invariably confronted with problems that on their face

---

2 Jim Carlton. "Compaq PCs Outsold IBM and Apple World-Wide During the First Quarter." *The Wall Street Journal* (May 25, 1994): A3.

3 Kenichi Ohmae. *The Mind of the Strategist: Business Planning for Competitive Advantage* (New York: Penguin, 1983).

appear to be a certain way. The initial response might be to cut costs, increase the marketing budget, or revise some feature of the product. However rational or justified such responses might seem, from Ohmae's standpoint they are misguided because they are predicated on appearances, not underlying relationships. Like the experienced detective, Ohmae understands that things are not always as they appear.

Alternatively, Ohmae suggests dissecting problems into their constituent parts and then, having discovered their significance, reassembling them in such a way as to maximize competitive advantage. "In strategic thinking, one first seeks a clear understanding of the particular character of each element of the situation and then . . . restructure(s) the elements in the most advantageous way. . . . True strategic thinking thus contrasts sharply with the conventional mechanical systems approach based on linear thinking. But it also contrasts with the approach that stakes everything on intuition. . . . " For Ohmae, superior strategic thinking combines "rational analysis" with "imaginative reintegration" (12–15).

Asking questions is central to the art of strategic thinking. Too often, though, according to Ohmae, "*questions are not framed to point toward a solution; rather, they are directed to finding remedies to symptoms*" (15–16). Ohmae's distinction between symptoms and solutions follows from his insistence that strategic thinking should focus on underlying relationships as opposed to facts as they appear. Much of what he means by the art of strategic thinking involves sifting through, beneath, and around myriad empirical details to find the underlying relationships of a problem. Those relationships, Ohmae emphasizes, point to the critical business issues. Strategic thinking that focuses on appearances vindicates preconceived notions and clouds the search for critical issues. Strategic thinking that goes beneath appearances to underlying relationships seeks the nature of the problem— for it is in the nature of the problem that there lies the solution.[4]

Though these points are not altogether explicit, Ohmae suggests a four-step "abstraction process" for identifying critical issues and solutions:

---

[4] This particular insight owes much to my many conversations with Hal Adams, a futurist, in Los Angeles, California.

❑ List all of the concrete factors in which a business is at a disadvantage relative to its competition.

❑ Group these factors into discrete categories based on some common denominator or principle that each group shares.

❑ Evaluate the underlying relationships in each discrete category to identify the critical issue.

❑ Ask solution-oriented questions of each group's critical issue, translate these solutions into concrete actions, and then prioritize these actions based on what is most important or strategic for the business.

Ohmae adds substance to this abstraction process by drawing on his engineering background and introducing two concepts the strategist can use in evaluating competing products: value engineering and value analysis. Value engineering helps determine if "quality and reliability are right for a particular product design and function." Value analysis helps determine if a product's "costs are reasonable for the product price" (23). He incorporates both value engineering and value analysis in two very useful exercises for identifying critical issues and asking solution-oriented questions. These exercises are presented in Figure 2–1 and Figure 2–2.

In a spirit reminiscent of Tregoe and Zimmerman, Ohmae suggests that companies too often short circuit the abstraction process in formulating strategy. By doing so, they abandon the art of strategic thinking. It is just this tendency that promotes the routinization of strategy described in the last chapter.

THE ART OF STRATEGY IN HEALTHCARE

Some time ago, I helped develop a new strategy for the full-time faculty of one department in a major medical school. Academic faculty practices generally are behind the marketplace, and this was certainly the case here. In theory, a clinical faculty's great strength is the prestige that differentiates academic physicians from competing physicians in the community: Academic physicians are the experts community physicians turn to. In practice, however, academic physicians are often locked out of referrals because of competition from the growing number of fellowship trained specialists and subspecialists practicing in the community. Indeed, one question residency

Figure 2–1.   A Sample Issue Diagram

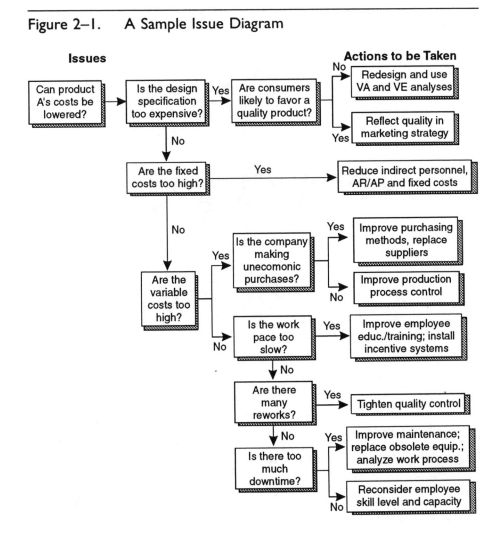

Source: Kenichi Ohmae. *The Mind of the Strategist* (New York: Penguin, 1983). Reproduced with permission of McGraw-Hill, Inc.

and fellowship programs often consciously address in selecting candidates for their programs is how much future competition faculty members are willing to produce.

My client faced not only these standard problems, but a host of others as well. As a result, they were not getting the referrals they needed. This impacted the department both financially and clinically, since faculty members who were not seeing a substantial number of tertiary cases were not generat-

Figure 2–2.   Product Change Options

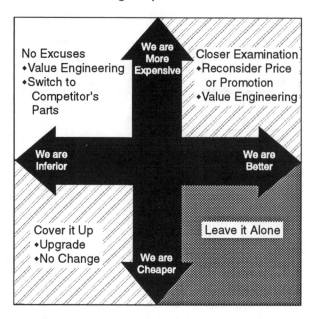

Source: Kenichi Ohmae. *The Mind of the Strategist* (New York: Penguin, 1983). Reproduced with permission of McGraw-Hill, Inc.

ing adequate revenues nor honing their special skills. We were brought in specifically to increase the department's tertiary referrals.

During the course of the engagement, three faculty members pressured us to approve a proposal to start their own satellite in an upscale community far removed from the department's service area. Other faculty members pressured us to formalize a referral arrangement with a local medical group known for being a "mill" because of their high volume and mixed results. Another faculty member wanted our advice for a new satellite office he intended to open in the prestigious downtown area. Still another wanted us to market a satellite office he had established near his home. And yet another faculty member, who was spending at least half his time in private practice deep in the department's secondary service area, wanted us to argue for the department picking up part of his overhead.

Taking a page from Ohmae, I decided not to focus on any of these "solutions," even though they all had the potential to increase department referrals somewhat. My concern was that they had a far greater potential to splinter the department and further weaken its position in the marketplace. After we conducted a series of interviews as part of an overall internal and external assessment, we identified an extensive list of problems, each of which could be construed as critical.

The short list of problems included: 1) the department's location; 2) the mystique of downtown, where the public assumes all the best doctors practice; 3) competition from other major medical centers; 4) competition from fellowship-trained subspecialists in the community; 5) a terrible patient mix; 6) primary/tertiary distinctions not being clear-cut; 7) "town/gown" personality conflicts; 8) lack of support from the voluntary staff (community physicians with admitting privileges at the medical center); 9) the department's reputation being far too dependent on its chairman; 10) the department lacking strong ties to the major players and power bases in the market; 11) the department not receiving HMO referrals; 12) scheduling, equipment, and staffing problems with the operating room; 13) deficient patient processing; 14) an inadequate and poorly motivated administrative staff; and 15) a scholasticism among some of the full-time faculty, to the point where they lacked the basic skills necessary to market themselves to referring physicians.

After identifying these problems, we clustered them into categories and then generalized from those categories to what we felt the critical issues were. As shown in Figure 2–3, we concluded that the department had five critical issues: 1) isolation, 2) perception, 3) two forms of competition, 4) operations, and 5) product definition. From there we identified two core strategic implications: 1) develop a new market position; and 2) improve operations, staff development, and product line management. Though both strategic implications were important, it was our belief that changing the department's market position should have priority. This abstraction process is presented in Figure 2–3.

At this point, the key question became, What will it take to change the department's market position? Our answer was that the department should:

- ❑ Adopt a very specific satellite strategy;
- ❑ Pursue a series of high-tech initiatives;
- ❑ Establish selective community-based/faculty alliances; and
- ❑ Implement high-profile public relations activities.

Figure 2–3.   Critical Issues and Strategic Implications

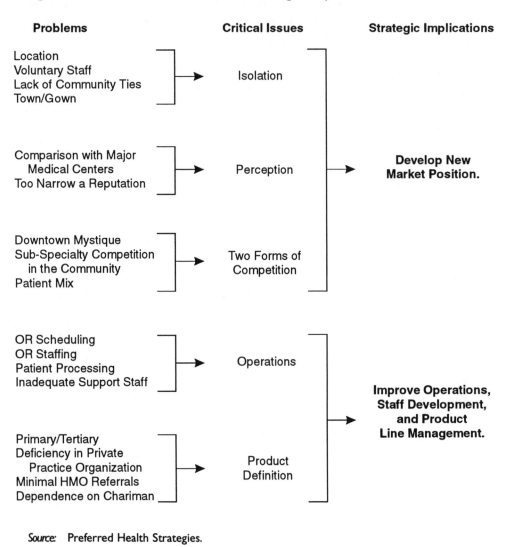

Problems	Critical Issues	Strategic Implications
Location Voluntary Staff Lack of Community Ties Town/Gown	Isolation	Develop New Market Position.
Comparison with Major Medical Centers Too Narrow a Reputation	Perception	
Downtown Mystique Sub-Specialty Competition in the Community Patient Mix	Two Forms of Competition	
OR Scheduling OR Staffing Patient Processing Inadequate Support Staff	Operations	Improve Operations, Staff Development, and Product Line Management.
Primary/Tertiary Deficiency in Private Practice Organization Minimal HMO Referrals Dependence on Chariman	Product Definition	

Source: Preferred Health Strategies.

Fortunately, the chairman accepted these recommendations, and the department began to turn itself around. I am convinced that if we had encouraged all of the separate initiatives that had been brewing in the department among individual faculty members, things would have gotten a lot worse. While it is not uncommon for businesses and organizations in the health-care industry to fail, it is unlikely that failure occurs before management has a chance to change direction. In most instances, I suspect, management has the opportunity to change direction, but too quickly accepts the facts as they appear, facts that justify actions that cannot stop the eventual decline.

COMPETITIVE ADVANTAGE AS STRATEGIC ADVANTAGE

Like Tregoe and Zimmerman, Ohmae distinguishes between strategic planning and the kind of planning required to achieve operational improvements. "What business strategy is all about—what distinguishes it from all other kinds of business planning is, in a word, *competitive* advantage" (36). Ohmae makes this distinction to emphasize two very special points:

❏ First, there is an enormous difference between strategic and operational issues from the standpoint of urgency. "Internal weaknesses or inefficiencies can usually be tolerated, at least for a time. By contrast, deterioration of a company's position relative to that of its competitors may endanger the very existence of the enterprise" (37).

❏ Second, strategic thinking "requires a very specific type of thinking. When one is striving to achieve or maintain a position of relative superiority over a dangerous competitor, the mind functions very differently from the way it does when the object is to make internal improvements with reference to some absolute model. It is the difference between going into battle and going on a diet" (37).

In business, Ohmae cautions, "perfect" strategies are not necessary. What counts is not strategy as measured against some absolute standard, but strategy that enables one business to gain a sustainable advantage relative to competitors. "A good business strategy, then, is one by which a company can gain significant ground on its competitors at an acceptable cost to itself" (37–38).

Here, Ohmae's Japanese perspective is particularly instructive. Since the resource limitations of this island country created a relatively low threshold of acceptable cost, Japanese businesses competing against larger U.S. and European firms have been forced to choose their battlefield carefully. A key element in the Japanese approach is to avoid head-on competition against a more formidable player, to choose the battlefield carefully and, if at all possible, to change the battlefield (240–241).

Most businesses, Ohmae argues, never engage in this kind of strategic thinking. "Their competitive posture is reactive 'If my competitor does it, I'll do it. If he attacks, I retaliate.' They don't try to develop a competitive differential. And that's a fatal error for anyone but a giant, because where there is no competitive differential, the giant will always win" (214).

ROUTES TO STRATEGIC ADVANTAGE

One goal of strategic thinking should be to gain, as efficiently as possible, a sustainable edge over competitors. Ohmae is certainly not the only strategist to make this point, but he may be one of the most eloquent. He describes four general ways in which strategic advantage can be achieved:

- ❏ Focusing on key factors for success;

- ❏ Building on relative superiority;

- ❏ Pursuing aggressive initiatives; and

- ❏ Exploiting strategic degrees of freedom.

These "routes to strategic advantage" are summarized below.

Focusing on Key Factors for Success

Every business has a finite amount of resources: capital, personnel, technology, and reputation. While allocating them in the same way as others accomplishes little, focusing them in a specific area that holds the key to success in an industry could well create a competitive advantage. By focusing on an industry's key factor, businesses can concentrate their resources to gain the upper hand. Even when a business has no more or better resources than its competitors, "it can achieve resounding competitive success if it is effective in bringing those resources to bear on the one crucial point" that exists in its industry (39).

Ohmae suggests two exercises for identifying the key factors for success: dissecting an industry as imaginatively as possible and analyzing the differences between winners and losers.[5]

---

5 The remainder of this section is drawn from Ohmae, 42–49.

❑ By dissecting an industry, he means analyzing its market segments. What are the major market segments and products? What are the major requirements of each market segment and product? It may be, for example, that most businesses are competing in one or more market segments that have a number of different requirements. The conclusion: Focus on that one segment, and concentrate your resources on that one requirement where success is most attainable. Or it may be that an emerging product feature is likely to have significant market appeal. The conclusion: If your competitors have tended to ignore this new feature, focus your resources to most effectively exploit it.

❑ To highlight the differences between winners and losers, Ohmae suggests comparing the key factors for success in generating profits and gaining market share across industries. He lists nine generic factors covering both upstream and downstream business functions. For illustration purposes, I have applied those factors to his discussion of the uranium and forklift truck industries illustrated in Figure 2–4:

Figure 2–4.   How Success Factors Vary by Industry

Key Factor in an Industry	Increase Profit	Increase Market Share
Raw material sourcing	Uranium	
Product facilities		
Design		
Production technology		
Product range		
Engineering		
Sales force		
Distribution network		Forklift
Servicing		

Source: Kenichi Ohmae, *The Mind of the Strategist* (New York: Penguin, 1983). Reproduced with permission of McGraw-Hill, Inc.

▪ Since the market price for uranium does not vary among producers, raw material sourcing is critical to profits in the uranium industry.

■ In the forklift industry, companies with distribution networks serving forklift and trucking customers do not have as much market share as companies with distribution networks serving forklift customers alone.

For businesses with competitors having equal or even superior resources, concentrating on one key factor may be the best opportunity for success. Businesses that do so and become good at it may then move to consolidate their leadership around other factors and build on their success. Businesses that either ignore their industry's key factor or are somehow ineffective in focusing on it are usually left behind.

Building on Relative Superiority[6]

Competitive advantage can still be achieved in situations when every competitor in the market is both aware of the key factor for success in their industry and focused on it. The challenge is to isolate some discrepancy in cost or function between two competitors and then build on that discrepancy to create a position of relative superiority. In seeking relative superiority, it is best to *adopt initiatives that either cannot be easily countered, take too much time to duplicate, or contradict some aspect of the competition's core business*. Ohmae offers two examples.

In one example, Companies A and B manufacture copiers. A's strategy is to price the small user at a loss since it is a "universal urge," as he puts it, for people working in office environments to copy everything in sight. A's profits are predicated on the small user eventually moving up to the higher end of its product line where the margins are greater. This strategy has been successful for years. Seeing this, B realizes that it cannot win over A's small users because the prices are too low. But it can price its products at the higher end far more competitively. Gradually, A loses its higher-end customers and has proportionately more business at the lower end where it is losing money. The more A reduces its prices at the higher end in retaliation, the less it can cross-subsidize its business at the lower end. As A and B slug it out, B's strategy based on relative superiority at the high end pushes A into a quagmire from which it cannot escape.

---

6 This section is drawn from Ohmae, 50–56.

In a second example, Companies A and B produce machinery. Where A had a more established operation in servicing, B had a stronger operation in sales. Because A's after-sales servicing was able to yield a far greater return than B's, A lowered its sales price, which B was immediately forced to match. Quickly, B found itself having to battle A on two fronts: depressed new machine prices and unprofitable service operations. In industries governed by fixed costs, one company will usually be at a significant disadvantage if its competitor is intent on exploiting the difference in cost structures between the two companies.

Pursuing Aggressive Initiatives[7]

Where the situation is either stalemated or declining, it is virtually impossible to bring about meaningful improvement by either working harder or trying to do better. Under those circumstances, what is called for according to Ohmae is "a thoroughgoing challenge to the accepted common sense of the industry." Here, the strategist should: 1) list the basic assumptions of the industry and ask whether they still apply; and 2) "confront what is taken for granted in an industry or business with the simple question, Why?" In the same way that great inventors owe their success to an inquisitive orientation, Ohmae insists that strategic thinkers can achieve comparable leaps of discovery that bear on business competition. He cites three Japanese examples:

- ❏ When a camera manufacturer asked why the nuisance of attaching a light fixture to a camera was necessary, his company developed a 35 mm camera with a built-in flash.

- ❏ When another camera company asked why there was always a vast discrepancy between exposed film and actual pictures taken, it discovered that people had difficulty loading their film. This caused the company to design an automatic loading mechanism for cameras.

- ❏ When the leader of Toyota Motor Company asked why his industry had to stockpile all of the components it needed for production, it led to the development of the "just-in-time" or *kanban* system and eventually to Toyota becoming a worldwide leader in automotive manufacturing.

---

7 This section is drawn from Ohmae, 57–61.

Exploiting Strategic Degrees of Freedom[8]

Ohmae's final route to strategic advantage involves his concept of strategic degrees of freedom. This refers to actions a business can potentially take vis-á-vis the "objective functions" in an industry.

The objective function is the value of a product or service considered most important in the customer's mind. Inherent in the objective function are "axes," with each axis consisting of a series of variables. These axes and their subordinate variables produce the desired value customers relate to. In exploiting a business's strategic degrees of freedom, the strategist looks for one or more axes where it would be most advantageous to concentrate. That choice should be made after careful analysis: 1) whether and under what circumstances the user's objective function will change; 2) short- and long-term technological factors; 3) development time; 4) the point when diminishing returns set in; and 5) competitor issues, including the anticipated market response.

In Ohmae's example, a camera manufacturer serves the amateur photography market. The objective function in that market is to get consistently good quality pictures at a reasonable cost. Strategic thinking calls for identifying the degrees of freedom—or axes—responsible for the consumer's major concern. As illustrated in Figure 2–5, Ohmae identifies seven different degrees of freedom.

By analyzing each axis, it is possible to evaluate a series of distinctive strategies. Ohmae then suggests that, because technological prowess is a mainstay of this manufacturer, the business should concentrate on three axes or degrees of freedom out of the original seven. The three are displayed in Figure 2–6.

For Ohmae, exploitation of strategic degrees of freedom is not something to be done quickly or intuitively. Axes should first be identified, then detailed, and finally evaluated. While evaluation has to take profits into consideration, the central issue is whether exploiting degrees of freedom around a specific objective function will lead to strategic advantage in the marketplace.

---

8 This section is drawn from Ohmae, 62–75.

Figure 2–5.   Strategic Degrees of Freedom for Improving Quality
of Finished Photographs

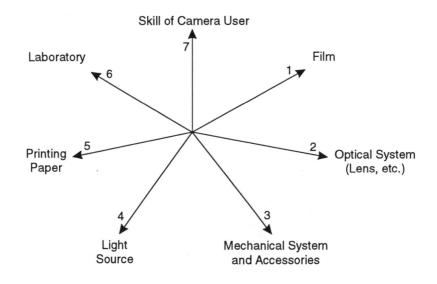

Source: Reprinted from Kenichi Ohmae, *The Mind of the Strategist* (New York: Penguin, 1983). Reproduced with permission of McGraw-Hill, Inc.

ROUTES TO STRATEGIC ADVANTAGE IN HEALTHCARE

Ohmae's routes to strategic advantage can be illustrated by two examples in the healthcare industry. The first involves the now defunct Humana hospital system. Humana viewed horizontal integration through HMO development as the best bet for the long-term success of its business. HMOs were embraced because of their capacity to direct or channel patients to Humana hospitals. This is a failure story, however, because Humana's management did not completely appreciate the underlying relationships associated with HMOs and their participating hospitals. Management did not grasp, in Ohmae's terms, the "strategic degrees of freedom" which had to fit just so if the strategy was to be successful.

Figure 2–6.   Three Selected Degrees of Strategic Freedom

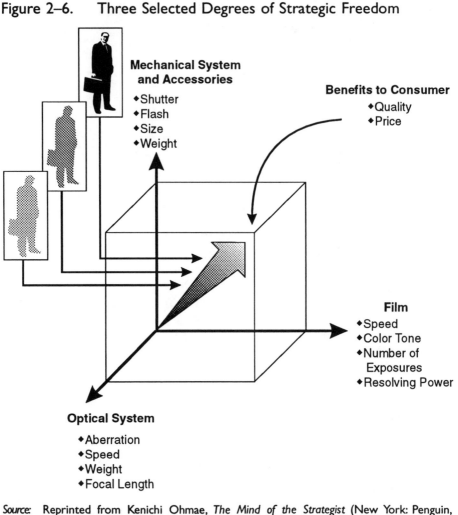

Source: Reprinted from Kenichi Ohmae, *The Mind of the Strategist* (New York: Penguin, 1983). Reproduced with permission of McGraw-Hill, Inc.

Management decided that HMOs should be the linchpin to its insurance strategy. HMOs would provide the vehicle for capturing an insured population and then channeling patients to the system's hospitals. In adopting this strategy, management created a separate division responsible for HMO development. Now the company had essentially two core businesses—hospitals and HMOs—with each expected to make a profit by supporting the other. It was considered a "brilliant strategy." "Perfect synergy." Even Wall Street applauded. One thing was forgotten, though: analysis!

If management had analyzed the situation, it would have recognized three critical weaknesses: 1) competing HMOs would now be less motivated to use Humana hospitals; 2) physicians not in the Humana Health Plan had no special reason for referring patients to Humana hospitals; and 3) Humana Health Plan physicians, unless pressured otherwise, could just as easily send their members to a participating non-Humana facility as a Humana facility.

Eventually, hospital admissions as well as HMO enrollments declined, and the two divisions experienced heavy losses. In addition, the company was forced to compete on two very different battlefields: with HMO and hospital competitors each having clear cut business objectives as well as the ability to effectively concentrate their resources. After numerous salvage attempts, hundreds upon hundreds of millions of dollars in losses, and considerable bad press because of a series of questionable business practices, Humana was split into two entirely separate companies, each intent on going in its own direction. The hospitals were spun off as Galen Healthcare, with Galen itself since being absorbed by a larger hospital corporation.[9] As for Humana Health Plan, it is now a large regional player with no special strengths, physician support, or member loyalty.[10] Such is the unique path to strategic advantage for much of American medicine in its "competitive era."

---

[9] It is more than a little ironic that management, in spinning off of the original Humana hospital system, chose the name Galen. While Galen is one of the most famous names in medical history, his fame does not stem from any positive clinical achievement. It stems from the fact that his writings were the last link in the continuum of ancient Greek and Roman medical literature and that they were translated, retranslated, and adopted as medical gospel for almost 1500 years. Galen actually represents the darkest moment in medical history because his writings were appropriated by the Church and used to integrate Christian teleology into the logic of medical practice throughout the Middle Ages. In fact, medicine not only did not, but epistemologically could not, begin to become an empirical science until the mantle of Galen was removed from medical education during the Renaissance.

[10] And, I would add, no special claim to providing a consistently high level of quality to its members. Humana's Florida Gold Plus Plan, for example, was recently denied accreditation by the National Committee for Quality Assurance (NCQA), the managed care industry's oversight group. The Gold Plus Plan is Humana's largest and most important HMO in Florida, serving approximately 217,000 Medicare members. See, "Humana Denied Accreditation for HMO in South Florida." *Sun-Sentinel* (August 16, 1994): 6A; and Louise Kertesz. "Humana Florida HMO Denied Accreditation." *Modern Healthcare* (August 22, 1994): 6.

A second example is the complete opposite. This situation involves a single physician who practices in an extremely competitive market. The market is distinguished by a disproportionately large Medicare population and by very significant managed care penetration. If you were to project the current situation forward, the picture would not be pretty for most physicians: cutthroat competition, constraints on specialty referrals, reduced reimbursement, and increased bureaucratic control on the everyday practice of medicine. While the characteristics of this particular market are somewhat unusual, the frustrations physicians feel there are similar to the frustrations of many physicians throughout the country.

The typical physician response is reactive. Physicians will start a new satellite. They will buy fancy new equipment. They will advertise. They will try to develop a reputation in some "hot" new procedure. Some will panic. Some, at the peak of their craft, will simply sell out. Some will put the squeeze on their pharmaceutical and equipment reps for kickbacks. And some will perform additional tests and procedures to compensate for cuts in reimbursement.

The situation I am describing is a success story, however, because the physician in question did not look to "game" the system. Instead, he sought to develop a strategic advantage by leveraging the unique resource physicians still have in the marketplace—control over clinical decision making.

The physician saw that HMOs were capitating medical groups and IPAs. These organizations, in turn, consisted of participating providers who agreed to treat HMO members at a discount. This particular physician took the IPA concept one step further and created his own specialty IPA network. The network was developed to cover a broad service area and to include all the subspecialists needed for most conceivable conditions in this one specialty. With the network in place, the physician contracted with the major HMOs to be the exclusive provider of services for his specialty. Now he received the capitation, paid his participating providers and, with them, established a quality assurance program consistent with their professional values. He also eliminated much of the HMOs' bureaucratic controls that represented nuisance costs to physicians. The HMOs were pleased because they could shift the risk to physicians who are in the best position to weigh the costs and benefits of clinical decisions. And the physicians were pleased because they could practice medicine under conditions they once again controlled.

This case represents a success story because of the way this physician sought to establish his strategic advantage. He understood that the basic role of the physician had not changed, but that a key factor for success in today's managed care marketplace had. Physicians can no longer position themselves individually vis-á-vis managed care systems. Now they have to position themselves institutionally. Individually, physicians have no countervailing power relative to the larger insurance companies and HMOs, but institutionally they can function on a level playing field. By forming his own network, he shifted the battleground in such a way that physicians could leverage their unique role to achieve a strategic advantage, rather than compromise their role for narrow, personal gain.

These two stories differ not just in the quality of strategic thinking each demonstrates, but in the way responsibility informed the pursuit of strategic advantage. In the first instance, a major corporation with considerable resources thought it was thinking strategically, when in fact it was just gambling. In the second instance, the single physician *had* to think strategically; he could not afford to gamble. In this sense, the difference between Humana and the physician also demonstrates a difference in business perspective reflected in Ohmae's work: The difference between a U.S. perspective on the one hand, and a Japanese perspective on the other.

STRATEGIC TRIANGLE

In formulating strategy, Ohmae maintains that three separate stakeholders need to be considered: 1) the customer, 2) the corporation, and 3) the competition. The job of the strategist is to identify the needs of the customer, properly match the strengths of the company with the customer's needs, and achieve superior performance relative to the competition. "A successful strategy is one that ensures a better or stronger matching of corporate strengths to customer needs than is provided by competitors" (91). For Ohmae, this tripartite relationship requires the integration of three different strategies: customer, corporate, and competitor based.

Customer-Based Strategies[11]

Customer-based strategies segment the market in two ways: by customer objectives and by customer coverage. Differences of age, sex, race, and income describe differences in the market, but according to Ohmae these are only "convenient statistical classes," not true segments. The strategist should distinguish among customer objectives to clearly understand differences in market segments. In addition to customer objectives, market segmentation involves understanding the trade-offs between marketing costs and coverage. Costs include promotion, sales, servicing, and distribution. These, in turn, all have to be weighed against the benefits of penetrating a specific market segment. The strategist's task is to optimize the range of market coverage so that the cost of targeting a market segment creates a competitive advantage.

Once market segments have been defined, they still need to be evaluated. In evaluating market segments, at least five separate industry trends should be considered: 1) trends in the structure of the market such as tendencies towards consolidation; 2) trends in user objectives and priorities; 3) trends in the customer mix; 4) trends in technology; and 5) trends in regulation. Any one of these trends, if it became dominant, could radically change the positives and negatives of a target market segment.

Corporate-Based Strategies[12]

As the outline of a customer-based strategy becomes clear, the strategist's perspective shifts to the company and the competition. Now the aim is to "maximize a corporation's strength relative to the competition in the functional areas that are critical to success in the industry" (110). For Ohmae, "functional areas" are the firepower companies bring to battle in the marketplace. They have to maintain a positive differential in a key functional area if they are to succeed.

It is in this context that Ohmae articulates one of the most intelligent long-term approaches to strategy formulation I am aware of: *sequencing improvement of functional competence*. "Sequencing" is distinguished from investing in numerous functional areas all at once. While the latter may lead to op-

---

[11]This section is drawn from Ohmae, 99–109.
[12]This section is drawn from Ohmae, 110–125.

erational improvements, it will not lead to a competitive advantage because no company can afford to invest in all key functions indefinitely. When a business gains a decisive edge in one functional area, it should then invest in a second area, gain an edge there, invest in a third area, gain an edge, and so on. Eventually, it will pull ahead of the competition.

According to Ohmae, the secret to many Japanese corporate success stories has been the ability to sequence improvement in key functional areas. Starting in the 1950s, for example, many Japanese companies focused initially on manufacturing engineering. Then they shifted their emphasis to quality control and product design. More recently, they have been active in basic research and direct marketing. The object of these functional strategies was not to solve operational problems, but to achieve a strategic advantage by strengthening specific functional performance.

Competitor-Based Strategies[13]

Competitor-based strategies represent the third leg of Ohmae's strategic triangle. Their focus is on differentiating one or more key business functions relative to the competition. Two themes stand out in Ohmae's discussion: "leakage analysis" and "tactics for flyweights."

As shown in Figure 2–7, leakage analysis enables the strategist to identify both the market segments that have been lost and the reasons why. The reasons could be because a product or service was not offered, certain customers were not covered, or customers have been competed for but lost to the competition. These reasons suggest possible areas in which a company might differentiate itself, which, in turn, suggest possible means of action. By identifying which segments are leaking, analyzing why, and then formulating a response, the strategist is in a position to create tangible differences in key functions between a company and its competition. To increase market share a company must first stop the leakage.

"Tactics for flyweights" is Ohmae's second theme that merits attention. Like the island nation of Japan, small players in the marketplace confront inherent disadvantages. Also, like Japan, small players can successfully take on the heavyweights by choosing to compete in ways the larger players cannot.

13This section is drawn from Ohmae, 126–135.

Figure 2–7.   Possible Sources of Competitive Differentiation

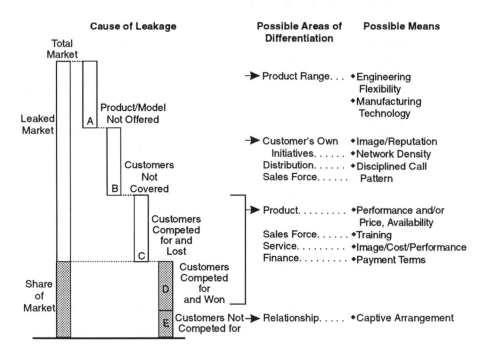

Source: Reprinted from Kenichi Ohmae, *The Mind of the Strategist* (New York: Penguin, 1983). Reproduced with permission of McGraw-Hill, Inc.

Ohmae cites as one example, Japan's top three home appliance makers who pay fixed incentives to dealers in strict proportion to sales. While a smaller competitor trying to outdo the big three on the same basis would never have the staying power to compete effectively, a smaller competitor could establish a variable incentive structure, offering dealers a graduated percentage and the potential for higher payments based on additional volume sold. Since the big three's profitability would soon be eroded if they offered their appliance dealers the same high percentages, the small appliance maker found an opening to exploit in the industry's distribution channels (134).

Even though larger companies have more resources, they are not immune from smaller competitors who pursue strategies that the larger company's size prevents. The trick is for the flyweight to take a different stance and compete against an aspect of the heavyweight's business that the heavyweight cannot respond to, usually because it contradicts some aspect of its core business. Such are the tactics of the flyweight.

STRATEGIC TRIANGLE IN HEALTHCARE

A few years ago, a hospital I am familiar with built a beautiful new facility to replace its main facility. The decision to undertake the rebuilding campaign was carefully considered. Since the hospital was located in a downtown area, one obvious issue was whether the area could support a new facility over the long term. The decision to move forward was based on projections that the downtown revitalization would continue. The expected growth of professional and white collar employees in the hospital's service area represented an attractive market the hospital assumed it could capture.

What stands out, in my judgment, was the mechanical and almost quixotic way in which hospital management went about its strategic thinking. The hospital explicitly projected 30 years into the future and committed itself to a long-term view at a time when projecting 5 years with any accuracy was hard enough. The 30-year time horizon justified the need for a replacement facility. It did nothing, however, to strengthen the quality of, or to inform, management's strategic thinking. Strategic thinking was driven by the pretense of being forward looking and innovative when, in fact, it was engaged in a crude, multimillion dollar wager. Unfortunately, this pattern appears all too often in our healthcare system.

As it turns out, the hospital has had an almost unbroken record of losing money, and the hospital system of which it is a part covers the loses. Ultimately, these loses are borne by all the citizens, businesses, and payors in the community. In addition, the hospital's management is under continuous pressure to "fix" the problem. Ironically, a new facility that was the result of a 30-year vision is now dependent on strategies that have a short-term, operational focus.

While this hospital is no different than any other hospital having to confront hard decisions about replacing an old facility, it is the presumptuousness of the 30-year vision coupled with the absence of any "sequential strategy" that is so telling.

Compare, for example, this hospital's strategic thinking to Honda Motor Corporation. In the early 1970s, the Honda Civic was a small, tinny car with little national appeal. Gradually, Honda engineered a variety of design and function changes and eventually incorporated them into the Honda Accord. By the mid-1980s the Accord became the top selling car in the United States. Not satisfied, Honda applied its same engineering and manufacturing prowess to develop a luxury car that could be priced below most Mercedes models. By the late 1980s, Honda's Acura was introduced. It quickly became a standard of excellence in the luxury car market, and neither Detroit nor the Germans have recovered.

There is nothing intrinsic to the healthcare industry that prevents hospitals, or for that matter, insurance companies and physicians, from following the path that Honda took: excelling in one functional area, competing successfully, and then extending that success to other functional areas and markets a step at a time. However, there is a tendency for business thinking in medicine to be conditioned by the same *hubris* that exists in medicine itself. Just as medicine assumes a cause and effect logic of intervention and cure, much of the business thinking that goes into medicine assumes a cause and effect logic of investment and success. Whether it be competitive forces, industry trends, or unanticipated developments, though, the road from investment to success in the medical marketplace is hardly straightforward. While big-time investments are often made with the expectation that they will pay off, too often they don't. As the loses mount, there is a tendency to blame the system: an "imperfect market" or things being "too complex." Notwithstanding the system's problems, consistent business success in medicine is most likely to be achieved when strategic thinking first grasps the nature of the problem, maps a path from point A toward point B based on that understanding, and then moves forward sequentially following a clearly formulated route to strategic advantage. This, as opposed to strategic thinking which simply forges ahead from point A, naively assuming that point B will be reached.

CHAPTER 3

The Force of Strategy

Strategic thinking in corporate America has changed over the past two decades. Traditionally, it had been a top-down exercise, with strategy in the form of mission, goals, and objectives determined first. Once these were determined, actions followed. The assumption was that a desired future could be imposed on the marketplace. Now, strategic thinking tends increasingly to be from the bottom up. The marketplace is examined first, and then strategy is formulated. The assumption here is that business cannot simply impose its will on the marketplace. There has to be a fit. The change from a top-down to a bottom-up approach is evident in the healthcare industry as well. For business generally, this change reflects the successful penetration of Japanese and other foreign competitors into U.S. markets. For the healthcare industry, it reflects a shift from the more regulated environment of the 1950s, 1960s, and 1970s, to a more competitive environment in the period since.

Al Ries and Jack Trout have written a series of books that focus squarely on this newer orientation.[1] Central to their thinking is that business strategy should be modeled on warfare. While their books were written from the point of view of marketing, the principles they develop relate to business strategy as a whole. Where Ohmae stressed the connection between strategy and a competitive edge, Ries and Trout demonstrate *how that edge can be created* through what they call "marketing warfare." Their point of view is bold and creative, and has the capacity to push healthcare strategy in new and different ways.

FROM PRINCIPLES OF WAR TO PRINCIPLES OF STRATEGY

The classic definition of marketing strategy involves meeting customer needs. Firms conduct market research to build their strategies around exactly what customers need. General Motors, Ford, Chrysler, and all of the other car makers spend millions of dollars annually conducting market research. Ries and Trout ask: Is this what successful strategy is all about, doing a better job of market research? Their answer is no. Customer needs should not drive business strategy; competitors should. When American Motors came up with the Jeep, it ignored customer needs and hit on a small niche competitors ignored. If American Motors remained focused on Jeeps, it might still be in business. But it used profits from Jeep sales to improve passenger cars, presumably to better satisfy customer needs. The subsequent difficulties American Motors encountered were not with its customers, though. They were with competitors such as General Motors, Ford, Honda, and Toyota (1986, 2–3).

Business success today requires that strategy be competitor oriented. The strategist "must look for weak points in the positions of competitors and then launch marketing attacks against those weak points" (1986, 4–5). Aggressiveness, especially aggressiveness distinguished by what the authors call the "more school of management," is not the sign of a winning strategy.

---

[1] Al Ries and Jack Trout. *Positioning: The Battle for Your Mind* (New York: Warner Books, 1981); Al Ries and Jack Trout. *Marketing Warfare* (New York: McGraw Hill, 1986); and Al Ries and Jack Trout. *Bottom-Up Marketing* (New York: McGraw Hill, 1990).

"Whenever you hear a commander say, 'We have to redouble our efforts,' you know you are listening to a loser" (40–41). Much better are efforts predicated on some kind of mismatch. For Ries and Trout, *mismatches can be created* if those who shape business strategy follow certain basic principles of war. Two principles drawn from the great Prussian general, Clausewitz, receive particular attention:

- ❏ **Principle # 1: The Principle of Force.**[2] "No other principle of warfare is as fundamental as the principle of force. . . . The big fish eat the small fish. The big company beats the small company." Paraphrasing Ries and Trout: When two companies go head to head, God smiles on the bigger company. If big beats small, do the weak ever have a chance? For the authors, the answer is yes—if they have a superior strategy. Quoting Napoleon, they suggest that his criteria for superior strategy in military campaigns applies to marketing as well: "The art of war with a numerically inferior army consists in always having larger forces than the enemy at the *point which is to be attacked or defended.*"

- ❏ **Principle # 2: The Superiority of the Defense.**[3] "Throughout military history, defense has proved to be the stronger form of warfare." Similarly with business. "If you can win the marketing battle and become the leading brand in a given category, you can enjoy that victory for a long time." Ries and Trout cite a survey of 25 leading brands from 1923. "Sixty years later, 20 of those brands were still in first place. Four were in second place and one was in fifth place." Competing against market leaders is not easy. "Ivory in soap, Campbell in soup, Coca-Cola in soft drinks. These represent strong marketing positions which can be taken only at great expense and with great energy." The main reason defensive warfare is so effective involves the difficulty of launching a surprise attack on those who already command the high ground. As a rule, leaders only lose if they ignore the signs of an enemy's attack, or if they think they are so big they don't have to defend themselves. When a market leader knows an attack is coming, the battle becomes a war of attrition. Under those circumstances, the mathematics always favor market leaders because of their ability to direct superior resources at the

---

2 This section is drawn from Ries and Trout, 23–29.
3 This section is drawn from Ries and Trout, 31–36.

point of attack—through advertising, service, rebates, price reductions, packaging, or whatever else it takes.

In formulating business strategy, the terrain is all-important. But where is the terrain? "Where are the marketing battles being fought?" They are not fought in supermarkets, boutiques, car dealerships, or shopping malls, the authors argue. Nor are they fought in places like New York, Chicago, Dallas, or Denver. They are fought in the mind of the consumer. They are fought on "mental mountains," where market recognition and brand identity exist (1986, 43–44). Mental mountains are created by 1) being first in the mind of the consumer; 2) having a clear and indelible message cut through our overcommunicated society; and 3) establishing an effective market position (1981, 1–51). Mental mountains are the icons of the marketplace, and they are fought over every day. Those sitting on top of the mountain invariably have a choice: Extend to protect the entire territory or contract to protect the home base. Extending is potentially very dangerous, the authors warn, because of the number of fronts that may have to be defended. "He who attempts to defend everywhere, defends nothing" (1986, 46–47).

The principle of force. The superiority of defense. Control of mental mountains. On the face of it, it would seem that winning and losing in the marketplace is almost preordained. For Ries and Trout, nothing could be further from the truth. Strategy *can* alter the conditions of combat and hence the conditions favoring one competitor over another. A tool the authors developed to accomplish that is what they call the "strategic square."

THE STRATEGIC SQUARE

"There is no one way to fight a marketing war. Rather there are four. [K]nowing which type of warfare to fight is the first and most important decision you can make."[4] Ries and Trout use the "big four" automakers in the early 1980s to illustrate the four different strategies competitors can choose from. General Motors, Ford, Chrysler, and American Motors were all significantly different in terms of strength and resources. "It's as if a grade school, a high school, a college and a professional football team were assem-

---

[4] This section is drawn from Ries and Trout, 49–54.

bled in a four-team league. Is there any doubt who would win?" But, the authors emphasize, "the game is more than winning." Because their circumstances are different, their strategies should be different as well:

- ❏ Since "General Motors will put more points on the scoreboard," GM wins simply by not losing. GM, in other words, should fight a *defensive war*.

- ❏ For Ford, increasing market share is the key to victory. Since Ford has the resources to capture additional market share, it should "attack GM because that's where the market is." Taking 10 percent from GM translates into a lot more business than taking 10 percent from Chrysler. Ford's best strategy is to launch an *offensive war* against the weak points in GM.

- ❏ For Chrysler, victory rests with "profitable survival." Rather than being drawn into the battle between GM and Ford, Chrysler's strategy should be to initiate a *flanking attack*, which is exactly what Lee Iacocca did with three separate products: The Chrysler convertible, the industry's first minivan, and the industry's first six-passenger, front-wheel drive car.

- ❏ For American Motors, victory is in surviving. American Motors was too small to have anything to really defend—too small to attack GM, Ford, or Chrysler, and too small to launch a flanking attack against the industry. What could American Motors do? Conduct a *guerrilla war* by targeting a segment big enough to be profitable, but small enough so as not to become the target of others. Having done this and succeeding with the Jeep, however, management forgot it was still limited to fighting only a guerrilla war.

The principles governing each of these four strategies are described in more detail below.

Principles of Defensive Warfare[5]

Ries and Trout list three principles of defensive warfare. Principle # 1 is that *defensive strategies should only be adopted by market leaders*. Those who adopt

---

5 This section is drawn from Ries and Trout, 1986, 55–66.

a defensive strategy thinking they are market leaders but in fact are not preempt future growth by limiting themselves to defensive moves.

Principle # 2 is that *the best defensive strategy is attacking yourself.* By introducing new products and services that make your existing ones obsolete; by taking business away from yourself before your competitors do; and by protecting your market share, even at the risk of sacrificing short-term profits.[6]

Defensive principle # 3 is that leaders should *always block strong competitive moves.* That could mean copying a competitor. It could mean striking back with lower prices. It could mean keeping something in reserve for massive advertising at a crucial point. Or it could mean seeking peace within the industry. If and when peace does break out, the market leader should shift from a brand emphasis to a generic emphasis: Campbell expanding the soup market, Kodak expanding the film market, and Microsoft expanding the software market. At this point, increasing the size of the pie becomes more profitable than increasing your slice of the pie.

Principles of Offensive Warfare[7]

There are no good strategies in theory. Good strategies depend on who specifically is using them. A good strategy for No. 1 in a market is not good for No. 2, and vice versa. Leaders should pursue defensive strategies; No. 2 and 3 should pursue offensive strategies.

Offensive principle # 1 is to *focus on the leader's strength.* Too often, Ries and Trout point out, companies focus on their own strengths, talking and acting as if they were the market leader but never becoming one. "No matter how strong a No. 2 company is in a certain category or attribute, it cannot win if this is also where the leader is strong." To successfully compete against the leader, it is not enough to succeed; you have to make the leader fail.

---

6 See, for example, Joan Rigdon. "Cannibalism Is a Virtue in Computer Business, Tandem's CEO Learns." *The Wall Street Journal* (August 24, 1994): A1. Referred to as "cannibalism" in this article, the *Journal* article describes how Tandem Computers, a leader in high-end mainframes, gutted its existing product line and introduced a lower-cost alternative. Quoting the head of Hewlett-Packard's computer business on this subject: "When you are at the top, you have to have the courage to say, 'I have to stop investing in this great product, and I'm going to use the money to generate a new product that will kill it.'"

7 This section is drawn from Ries and Trout, 1986, 67–81.

Offensive principle # 2 is to *identify a weakness in the leader's strength and attack that weakness*. Attack the weakness *in* the strength. "Rent from Avis. The line at our counter is shorter." This is one example the authors cite. Another is any No. 2 player who competes against a volume leader based on service—particularly if the volume leader produces an inferior product. Since the greater the volume, the greater the demand for service, with No. 1 diverting more energy and resources to service, No. 2 is in a much stronger position to challenge No. 1.

Offensive principle # 3 is to *pursue as narrow a line of attack as possible*.[8] That means with one product or one message or one initiative. Businesses who think they don't have the "luxury" of passing up larger opportunities miss the point. Trying to do it all—to sell multiple products across a variety of segments or to attack on multiple fronts—dilutes strength. Businesses falling into this trap are not only likely to lose in the long run, they are likely to lose a lot more than they ever gained.

Principles of Flanking Warfare[9]

Flanking is the prescribed strategy for No. 3 in a market. It is an offensive move that involves circumventing the industry's tacit knowledge. Flanking principle # 1 is to *target uncontested areas in the marketplace*. Digital flanked IBM with the minicomputer. Sun Computer flanked Digital with the workstation. Successful flanking depends on creating and maintaining a separate market territory, which is different than segmentation. "To launch a true flanking attack, you must be first to occupy the segment. Otherwise it's just an offensive attack against a defended position." Successful flanking also requires considerable foresight because there is no demonstrable market for the product or service as yet. Miller Brewing Company showed such foresight when it flanked the industry with Miller Lite.

Flanking principle # 2 is to *use tactical surprise*. The bigger the surprise, the bigger the opportunity to establish brand identity. Surprise can also demoralize competitors—by catching them flat-footed or tied up in other areas.

---

8 This point is consistent with Ohmae's concept of a sequential strategy. Attack narrowly, succeed, expand, and build further on your success.

9 This section is drawn from Ries and Trout, 1986, 83–99.

Flanking principle # 3 is to *continuously reinforce and strengthen the attack.* This is the "pour-it-on principle." Too many companies ignore this principle by taking profits from their success and investing it in other areas. When you have a flanking product that is not successful, drop it. When you are successful, invest heavily to strengthen your position before competitors can mount a challenge.

There are many different flanking moves. You can flank with a low price as Budget did or with a high price as Grand Union did with the Food Emporium. You can flank with a small size such as Volkswagon's Beetle or with a large size such as the Head tennis racket. Timex flanked successfully by using drug stores as a distribution system for selling watches. Perhaps the best example of a distribution flanking move is Hanes. When Hanes placed L'eggs in innovative packaging right next to supermarket checkout counters, sales for its panty hose took off. Companies that flank well substantially affect the availability of choices in the market. If they stay disciplined, they may eventually become market leaders.

Principles of Guerrilla Warfare[10]

In business as in war, size is important, but it is also relative. More important than your size is the size of your competitors. The smallest automotive company, Ries and Trout point out, is bigger than the largest textile manufacturer, but the automotive company should fight a guerrilla war and the textile manufacturer a defensive war. Guerrilla principle # 1 is to *target a market segment small enough to defend.* "A guerrilla organization does not change the mathematics of a marketing war. (The big company still beats the small company.) Rather, the guerrilla tries to reduce the size of the battleground in order to achieve a superiority of force." Successful guerrillas are "the big fish in the small pond." This is often achieved geographically— the local hotel being bigger and splashier than the Holiday Inn, or the local burger place being bigger and friendlier than the McDonald's. It is also achieved by product. Both Intel and Microsoft were once infinitely smaller than IBM. But they concentrated on products where their growth allowed them to defend themselves against the industry leader.

---

[10]This section is drawn from Ries and Trout, 1986, 101–116.

Guerrilla principle # 2 is *never act like the market leader, regardless of your success*. "[T]he essence of guerrilla strategy and tactics is the opposite of what's right for the Fortune 500 crowd." In Vietnam, the classic guerrilla war, the U.S. had a large proportion of soldiers in the bureaucracy, managing, supplying, and servicing the needs of the fighting soldiers. For the North Vietnamese, virtually every soldier had a gun on the firing line. It is the same with large corporations: Huge bureaucracies and a smaller percentage of the corporate army engaged in battle. "Guerrillas should exploit this weakness by getting as high a percentage of their personnel as possible on the firing line"—in marketing and sales.

Guerrilla principle # 3 is *be prepared to exit a market quickly*. If the product is not working, drop it. Large corporations cannot do that because there are too many higher ups with egos and jobs on the line. They stick with problems; guerrillas have the freedom to move on. Similarly with quick market entry. Large corporations require countless committee meetings to act on a hunch; guerrillas can act immediately.

Just as there are many different flanking attacks, there are many different guerrilla attacks. *Crain's* is a geographic guerrilla competing against *Business Week, Fortune,* and *Forbes*. Cuisinart is a high-end guerrilla competing against Sunbeam and GE. Apple was a product guerrilla until it became more of an industry leader. Most of America's corporations, the authors suggest, should be waging guerrilla warfare. "Out of every 100 corporations, as a glittering generality, one should play defense, two should play offense, three should flank, and 94 should be guerrillas."

STRATEGY AND TACTICS

Strategies are not successful because they are brilliant or different. They are successful because "they put troops in the field in exactly the right place and at the right time to accomplish the job tactically" (1986, 188). Strategies are only successful if they succeed tactically. The essence of a successful strategy, in other words, is successful tactics. One is not more important than the other. It is the relationship between the two that is important. "A tactic is a singular idea or angle. A strategy has many elements, all of which are focused on the tactic" (1990, 13). While a strategy unfolds over a period of time, a tactic unfolds at one time. Strategy formulation requires a critical understanding of how tactics can be expected to unfold in the heat of the battle.

For Ries and Trout, formulating the right strategy requires first finding the right tactic. "The tactic is the angle that produces the results. The strategy is the organization of the company to produce the maximum tactical pressure. . . . The tactic dictates the strategy. Then the strategy drives the tactic" (1990, 16). Within that framework, the authors make a series of points that bear on sound strategic thinking.

Going Down to the Front[11]

Three problems stand out with respect to much contemporary business strategy. First, market research focuses too much on the past. Research typically tells management what has been done, not where things are going. Second, those who set strategy are often removed from where the action is. They don't fully appreciate what is really going on in the marketplace. And third, when senior management does try to get close to the customer, it is usually with preconceived notions, rather than with an open mind. Going down to the front means senior management observing, not judging; seeking information, not confirmation; and, most importantly, looking for an angle in the marketplace, not simply "the answer."

Finding Your Tactic

For Ries and Trout, strategy formulation should "work from the specific to the general, from the short term to the long term." The specific is the tactic; the general is the strategy. "A tactic is external to the product, service or company. It need not even center on the product a company makes" (1990, 12). What's important is that the tactic yield some kind of decisive edge. In one instance, a single tactic might define strategy. For example, Domino's Pizza. "What made Domino's such a powerhouse were the strategic implications of the home delivery tactic" (1990, 14). In other instances, a series of tactics define strategy. For example, Apple Computer: Targeting the educational market; producing Newton, the first hand-held computer; aggressively lowering its prices to increase market share; and establishing separate

---

[11]This section is drawn from Ries and Trout, 1990, 18–38.

strategic alliances with Sony and IBM—all to support a strategy of extending Apple's reach throughout everyday life.

Finding the right tactic involves distinguishing trends from fads, and hype from reality. There are always popular ideas. But do they have staying power? Are they grounded in demographics, economics, and culture? Or are they just another fling in the marketplace? A pet rock or a swatch watch? A miniskirt or blue jeans? For the authors, the right tactic is in the long waves, 10-year trends, and underlying tendencies that may not get much press but evolve and endure.

Finding the right tactic also involves narrowing the focus. "Throughout history, battles were won because generals were able to concentrate their forces at the decisive point . . . they were able to focus their resources on a single sector of the front" (1990, 57). Too many companies, the authors warn, are fighting hundreds of brush fires rather than a single war. Simple ideas with a single thrust are invariably more successful than complex ideas with multiple thrusts. The right tactic is simple and singular. It allows for the concentration of resources, an effective message, and a clear brand identity.

Shifting the Battlefield

"At any given point in time, one objective should dominate a company's strategic plans" (1986, 196). Success with one objective, though, should not be separated from the strategy as a whole. Ries and Trout constantly stress the unity of tactics and strategy, the specific and the general. If the battle is to be won, it should not simply be for the sake of winning. It should be to support the larger strategy. If it is to be lost, then the battlefield should be shifted, but in a fashion consistent with tactics and strategy.

There are at least four ways to shift the battlefield:

❑ **Shift the Product.** Disney Studios, for example, tried unsuccessfully to produce movies that went beyond the industry's "G" rating. To correct this, they initiated a product shift by establishing Touchstone Pictures as a separate studio identified with adult movies. "The company now has two powerful entities: The Disney name and product for the family business and the Touchstone name for the adult business" (1990, 144).

❑ **Shift the Focus.** Shifting the focus means moving from a generalist to a specialist, sacrificing a part of the business to concentrate on a smaller part. At one time, Interstate Department Stores was a mediocre retailer, struggling in the discount wars. Interstate then bought a fledging Toys "R" Us and reorganized itself exclusively as a superstore for toys. Wall Street has celebrated this success story ever since (1990, 144–145).

❑ **Shift the Distribution.** You can shift the battlefield by shifting your distribution system. With a new distribution system, you have a new way to access customers (1990, 145–147). At the same time that Sears exited the mail-order catalog business, Saks Fifth Avenue and a number of other prominent retailers entered interactive home shopping cable ventures—a case of electronic distribution supplanting the more time-consuming mail-order format. Merck's acquisition of Medco, on the other hand, is tied to a mail-order tactic. Medco is the largest mail-order pharmaceutical distributor in the healthcare industry. By acquiring Medco, Merck shifted its distribution system from sales reps selling physicians to service contracts generating sales through HMOs and PPOs.[12]

❑ **Shift the Approach.** Shifting the approach turns on knowing what is fixed and what is variable in the market. If you can't change what is fixed, change your approach. If you can't change the mind of consumers, change your way into their mind. One way is to change your name. "Alphonso D'Abruzzo couldn't get a job on television until he changed his name to Alan Alda." Similarly, "Allegeny Airlines was going nowhere until it changed its name to USAir." Can Western Union ever make the transition to a high-tech information services company until it shakes its identity with the 19th century Pony Express? A second way is to change your price. In their home markets, Bally shoes (Switzerland) and Beefeater gin (England) are not the high-priced products they are in the United States. By adopting high prices in this country, though, both Bally and Beefeater were able to establish themselves at the premium end of the U.S. market. A third way is to change your business

---

[12]Elyse Tanouye. "Merck Will Exploit Medco's Data Base." *The Wall Street Journal* (August, 4, 1993): B1; and George Anders. "Managed Healthcare Jeopardizes Outlook for Drug 'Detailers.'" *The Wall Street Journal* (September 10, 1993): A1.

focus. Xerox, for example, tried in vain to become a force in the computer industry. Its problem, of course, was that to consumers Xerox meant copiers, not computers. Xerox did not reestablish itself as a growth company until it "changed" to being the leading copier company again (Ries and Trout, 1990, 123–132).

HMO WARS

HMOs will be discussed at length in subsequent chapters. Here it will suffice to say that the acronym stands for "health maintenance organizations," and that HMOs have been around for over four decades. Originally conceived to be total delivery systems consisting of hospitals, physicians, and the full continuum of ancillary services, HMOs did not really begin to have broad national appeal until the latter 1980s, in part because organized medicine resisted their growth; in part because consumers had been unwilling to accept limitations on their choice of providers; and in part because insurers did not push HMOs as a mainstream health insurance product. All of that has changed with the growing recognition that healthcare inflation is a serious national problem. Enter "managed care." Since the presidential election of 1992, it has become almost axiomatic that *managed care systems*, rather than doctor/patient transactions in a fee-for-service environment, should be the operative unit in healthcare delivery. With managed care systems organizing how health services are provided, the assumption is that cost containment will be achieved.

No system of managed care has been more widely touted as the cure for healthcare inflation than HMOs.[13] Frequent news coverage has educated the American public about how they work. National policy has embraced HMOs as an industry standard. And growing numbers of employers are actively encouraging their employees to select HMO coverage to keep healthcare costs down. In short, HMOs are no longer at the fringe of the product continuum. They represent more of the middle ground.

---

[13]See, for example, Peter Kerr. "The Changing Definition of Health Insurers." *New York Times* (May 10, 1993): D1; and Greg Steinmetz. "Clinton's Health Plans are Likely to Step Up the Switch to HMOs." *The Wall Street Journal* (May 18, 1993): A1.

Despite all of the positives surrounding HMO growth, however, there is an unmistakable "me too" tendency that informs HMO industry strategy. HMOs are falling all over one another copying their competitors at precisely the time they have their best opportunity to pursue different strategies *and* be successful. Recall Ries and Trout's general principle about strategy: There are no good strategies in theory. Good strategies depend on who specifically uses them. A good strategy for No. 1 in a market is not good for No. 2, and vice versa. Leaders should pursue defensive strategies; No. 2 and 3 should pursue offensive strategies. No. 4 and beyond should pursue guerrilla strategies. What is happening instead is that most HMOs are pursuing a standard vanilla strategy based on current industry thinking. In my judgment, this homogeneity detracts from the quality of medicine that HMOs are capable of providing. One example is the growing use of gatekeeper physicians by HMOs.

Gatekeepers[14]

At some point during the 1980s, an idea took hold in the HMO industry that every patient should have a primary care physician (PCP). The PCP's role was not just to serve as a patient's regular doctor, it was to coordinate his or her overall use of medical services. Thus, PCPs either provide the authorization for their HMO patients to see a specialist, or they seek authorization from the HMO's utilization review department. With the exception of emergencies, the same applies to hospitalization. In many instances, PCPs also authorize the use of laboratory and other diagnostic tests. For all intents and purposes, therefore, adoption of the gatekeeper/PCP role by HMOs has recast at least part of the family doctor's function from being strictly clinical, to *regulating* the services HMO members receive.

I see at least five problems inherent in the gatekeeper concept:

    ❑ First, most primary care physicians resent the policing qualities being a PCP requires. When patients call needing authorization, they either have to come in for a visit, clogging up the physician's already busy appointment schedule, or receive authorization over the telephone. If

---

[14]Though there are exceptions, these comments apply to almost all HMOs in the industry.

it is the latter, then serving as a gatekeeper really only exists for its sentinel effect. Since approval is usually given anyway, the sentinel effect is hardly a reason to make PCPs the foundation of the system.

❑ Second, the regulatory function in the gatekeeper role compromises the doctor-patient relationship. PCPs are evaluated by how many referrals they authorize, and how much the total utilization from those referrals actually cost. To the extent that PCPs keep the volume and costs associated with specialty referrals down, they are compensated additionally. To the extent that they don't, they not only lose money, their participation in the HMO could also be in jeopardy. For their part, if patients are having a medical problem they feel justifies a specialty referral, they make certain they get that referral . . . or they will leave the physician. As the author of a recent article on HMOs in New York put it: "Most of the doctors whom I interviewed told me they felt the gatekeeper role had strained doctor-patient relationships even further than they're already strained. That is ironic," she went on to say, "since HMOs aim to revive the role of the family doctor."[15]

❑ Third, by virtue of HMOs relying on private, independent physicians to do their bidding, there is a built-in tension between HMOs and PCPs that I do not believe can ever be resolved. The more HMOs try to regulate the clinical process through external controls, the more they will alienate the very producers they depend on. Physicians in private practice have chosen to be independent practitioners. Regardless of how inconsistent that goal may be in today's environment, the brute fact is that the goal and the requirements imposed by HMOs are contradictory. An internist, commenting in a *New York Times* Op-Ed article a few years back, summed it up well when he said, "Physicians feel increasingly beleaguered. Their recommendations and decisions are being questioned, constrained and overruled. Each third party payor is adopting policies to reduce its own reimbursement for care. Viewed narrowly, most of these cost reduction programs appear reasonable.

---

[15]Jeanne Kassler. "Managed Care—Or Chaos?" *New York Magazine* (August 23, 1993): 47. Also see Gina Kolata. "Wariness is Replacing Trust Between Healer and Patient." *New York Times* (February 20, 1990): A1.

The aggregate effect, however, is a bureaucratic maze that frustrates patients and providers alike—and doesn't save much money."[16]

❑ Fourth, while many PCPs have only a small percentage of their total patient base from any one HMO, their office staff has to contend with a disproportionate amount of bureaucracy and red tape. Stories of spending 20–30 minutes just on the telephone to obtain a single authorization abound in the industry. Besides the red tape, paperwork, and administrative costs, though, there is the issue of professional integrity. In situations where a very significant number of patients from one HMO comprise a PCP's practice, the PCP is beholden to the HMO. Under those circumstances, it is questionable whether HMO patients will receive their physician's best judgment if it conflicts with HMO medical policy. For example, a PCP with 1,500 patients might be paid a capitation of $10 per member per month, or $180,000 annually, from an HMO. As one doctor observed: "That's a lot of money for a physician to turn his back on if there's a difference of opinion between the doctor and the HMO" (Kassler, 49).

❑ Finally, the trend towards capitation does not eliminate the perverse incentive that has bedeviled the healthcare industry for decades. It simply reverses it. Now, rather than there being an incentive to do more, PCPs, as all physicians under capitation, have an incentive to do less. In addition to the perverse incentive affecting treatment, there is evidence that capitation causes dissatisfaction in the way patients feel they are being treated. This dissatisfaction is reflected in the mill-like quality of many large capitation practices.[17]

---

[16]Robert A. Berenson. "Meet Dr. Squeezed." *New York Times* (July 21, 1989): Op-Ed. There is no shortage of news coverage on this subject. See, for example, Lawrence Altman with Elisabeth Rosenthal. "Changes in Medicine Bring Pain to Healing Profession." *New York Times* (February 18, 1990): A1; Lisa Belkin. "Many in Medicine See Rules Sapping Profession's Morale." *New York Times* (February 19, 1990): A1; Lisa Belkin. "Doctors View Health Plans as Eroding Their Autonomy." *New York Times* (November 12, 1991): A1; and Ron Winslow. "Prescribing Decisions are Increasingly Made by the Cost Conscious." *The Wall Street Journal* (September 25, 1992): A1.

[17]See, for example, Ron Winslow. "Patients Prefer Small Providers of Healthcare." *The Wall Street Journal* (August 19, 1993): B1. This article refers to a study published that day in the *Journal of the American Medical Association*, which looked at 17,671 patients from 367 doctors in solo practice, large specialty groups, and HMOs in Boston, Chicago, and Los Angeles.

Notwithstanding problems with the gatekeeper/PCP role, the real danger in the HMO industry is that most refuse to buck the trend and pursue distinctive paths of development. Were some to do so, I'm convinced they would not only be better off, but the public would be as well. Instead, industry evolution is governed by the same basic gatekeeper logic. More than anything else, I believe, the recent upsurge in HMO enrollment can be attributed to an historic growth opportunity in the healthcare system, rather than to substantive differences in program or product where successful HMOs have achieved an edge over competitors.

Mechanical Strategy, Mechanical Performance

In Ries and Trout's thinking, there must be a unity between tactics and strategy, the specific and the general. The tactic should yield some kind of competitive advantage, and the strategy should sustain it. Finding the right tactic, they argue, involves distinguishing trends from fads and hype from reality. My own view is that the HMO industry's preoccupation with capitating PCP gatekeepers is a fad and that eventually it will exhaust itself.

Not long ago, I spoke with the medical director of a primary care group practice in Los Angeles. With over 40 percent HMO market penetration, Los Angeles is one of the largest HMO markets in the country. This medical director completely understood the significance of primary care physicians in an HMO dominated marketplace and that the PCP's role was central to how HMOs operate. His practice had a history of acquiring smaller primary care practices and had itself just merged with a much larger group practice. Their strategy was to consolidate operations under a single corporate entity to reduce overhead and capture as large a share of the region's HMO membership base as possible. When I asked him what kind of *clinical* efficiencies or changes in the medical division of labor they were considering, he had no answer. When I inquired how low- and high-tech equipment would be configured within the overall operation, he said no one had given it much thought. His point to me was that the group's physicians would continue to practice as they had in the past. Aside from eliminating administrative duplication and enjoying more effective group purchasing, there was no new approach or innovation planned that would enable his physicians to function more effectively under capitation.

While it is premature to say how things will turn out for this particular group practice (or others like it), my guess is that the future will not be positive. I say this for four reasons:

❑ **HMO Bargaining Power.** With few exceptions, it has been my experience that HMOs are absolutely committed to paying the least amount possible. Unless precluded from doing so, HMOs as a rule, would just as soon take their business elsewhere.[18] Those who assume larger group practices will balance the equation, forget the old adage that "He who pays the piper, calls the tune." Since large primary care practices are dependent on their gatekeeper contracts, the mere threat of an HMO backing away in a negotiation detracts from the practice's bargaining position. Should an HMO withdraw its business, it could have serious repercussions for a practice. I have seen group practices literally accept anything HMOs offer for fear of losing the business.

❑ **Inadequate Clinical Reorganization.** HMOs that capitate independent practitioners are in a structural dilemma: They set the budget for PCPs, but the PCPs have not changed their work flows, functions, tasks, and activities to operate under such budgets. It is one thing to assume that a doctor who was once paid based on charges can tolerate a 20–30 discount and still deliver a quality service to patients. It is quite another thing to take that same doctor, force him or her into a very tight fixed budget, and assume the same level of quality. I recognize the argument about capitation engendering discipline in medical practice. But *imposing fiscal discipline without bringing comparable innovations into the clinical process is a recipe for failure.*

❑ **HMO Requirements Exceeding MD/Vendor Status.** Though generally not referred to in these terms, PCPs, like all participating providers, are essentially vendors selling services to HMOs. To the extent that HMOs were not pressed to institute changes in the conduct of medical practice, the vendor relationship served the interests of the independent practitioner. Now, however, competitive pressures are forcing HMOs

---

18In most markets, there are more providers for an HMO to turn to than there are HMOs for the providers to turn to. Where there is a shortage of primary care physicians, HMOs can always recruit such doctors to develop satellite practices, or hire them—something growing numbers of HMOs are now beginning to do.

to be more aggressive in controlling costs. This suggests two problems. First, independent practitioners are not motivated to make the changes in medical practice that HMOs require. Second, the business goals of physicians in private practice are different than those of HMOs. As HMOs contend with the imperatives of competition, an aging population, and high-tech medicine, contradictory dynamics surrounding the physician/vendor relationship can be expected to become increasingly pronounced in the future.

❑ **Its the Specialists, Stupid.** The major source of HMO expenditures is at the specialty level. My impression from speaking with medical directors across the country is that specialty care as a whole generates about 70–75 percent of total medical expenditures.[19] In addition, the intensity and cost structure associated with specialty care is increasing much faster than primary care. Since the challenge is to control rising specialty costs, the question that has to be asked is why focus on primary care? The standard answer is that by limiting access to specialists through PCPs, you control specialty volume. Aside from burdening PCPs with the sins of the specialists, this approach prevents strategic thinking from focusing squarely on where the problem lies. The more HMOs focus on PCPs to control specialty care, the more neglected the specialty problem can be expected to become.

In the zero sum world of managed competition, the combined impact of these four factors leads inevitably, I believe, to an underlying mediocrity in the HMO industry: 1) HMOs bidding the price of primary care down, and PCPs having no choice but to accept what they're offered; 2) PCPs not being organized to achieve greater clinical efficiencies in the limited budgets they have to work with; 3) competitive pressures requiring HMOs to lean harder and harder on independent practitioners, straining already complicated vendor relationships; and 4) inflationary forces endemic to specialty care continuing unabated. Under these circumstances, a window of opportunity exists for those choosing to pursue something other than a gatekeeper/PCP strategy.

---

[19]Included in the category "specialty care" are specialists per se, specialty generated ancillary services, and hospital costs (inpatient as well as outpatient).

Lessons from the "Cola Wars"

With the HMO industry so unilaterally committed to a single basic model, how can one HMO differentiate itself from another? How can one gain an edge over another? Taking a page from Ries and Trout, one answer is to outflank the competition—circumventing an industry's tacit knowledge by targeting uncontested areas in the marketplace. But which uncontested areas? And how should they be targeted? Remember offensive principles # 1 and # 2: Focus on the leader's strength and attack the weakness in that strength. Ries and Trout's description of the Pepsi/Coke wars provides a case study in the application of these points to business strategy.

By the 1920s, Coca-Cola was the unmistakable leader among cola brands and enjoyed the dominant franchise in the soft drink market. Pepsi-Cola's first major move was as a small cola company battling the giant Coca-Cola. In the depression years, Coke was sold in 6 1/2-ounce bottles for a nickel. Coke management believed that its bottles were a major source of strength. They showcased the bottle in all their ads and even had it trademarked. One commentator called Coke's bottle, "the most perfectly designed package in use." So what did Pepsi do? It produced a 12-ounce bottle that sold for the same nickel. Combined with a catchy radio jingle, this strategy was an extremely effective flanking attack at the low end of the market. Pepsi attacked Coke's strength, turning the latter's strength into a weakness. The "perfectly designed 6 1/2-ounce bottle that fit the hand couldn't be scaled up to 12 ounces." Since Coke could not change its bottle, Pepsi caught on immediately with younger consumers who were sold on quantity rather than brand identity. In retrospect, Pepsi's strategy not only gave it a defined position in the cola market, it laid the foundation for future advertising campaigns based on the idea of a "Pepsi generation." By the end of World War II, Pepsi surpassed all but Coke, and became the established No. 2 in the market (1986, 119–121).

Flash forward. The "Pepsi Challenge" of the mid-1970s marked another significant move on Pepsi's part, for a time catapulting this perennial No. 2 company over Coke. In live, blind taste tests, Pepsi established the impression that it tastes better than Coke. Since Pepsi is about 9 percent sweeter than Coke, the promotion naturally favored Pepsi. Then Coke made a mistake. Rather than do what leaders should always do—block a strong competitive move—Coke retreated by changing its formula to match the sweetness of Pepsi. This turned out to be one of the great blunders in recent American business. It showed weakness. It confused the public. It alienated loyal Coke drinkers. And perhaps most importantly, it prevented Coke from claiming to be "the real thing" (1986, 133–134).

What is "the real thing"? For Coke, the real thing is a secrete formula dating back to the 19th century, a formula that supposedly only a handful of people have ever known. "The real thing" is mystique, tradition, and an uncompromised claim to being an American original, an American icon. When Coke changed its formula, Pepsi had in effect gotten Coke to change battlefields, to compete on Pepsi's terms. While sales figures point to Coke recapturing its No. 1 position, Coke now competes as a commodity, not as an icon. Once the genie is out of the bottle, you can never get it back in again.

Rethinking HMO Battle Plans

Consider the following. First, the public has always been concerned about the quality of specialty care in HMOs. Second, for serious problems, people tend to choose their specialists based on the reputation of the organizations they are associated with—Mayo Clinic, Yale, UCLA, Stanford, and so on. And third, a growing trend among HMOs is to link provider reimbursement to global budgets, be it capitation, case rates, or risk pools. Given these points, I think even the weakest of HMOs, if willing to buck current gatekeeper/PCP thinking, could effectively outflank their competitors in virtually any market in the country. The three moves outlined below represent one hypothetical flanking strategy:

❑ **Move# 1:** *Have as many primary care physicians on the HMO panel as possible, without gatekeepers and without capitation.* The key here is marketing: 1) give primary care the look and feel of the traditional middle-class system; 2) make it likely that when people choose an HMO, their primary care doctor will be a participating provider; and 3) ensure that HMO policies and procedures don't frustrate PCPs. While marketing is the major concern with move # 1, cost is not irrelevant. Physician monitoring, a discount fee schedule, reasonable withhold provisions, and patient co-payments of some substance should all be adopted. If patients insist on going to an HMO specialist without going through their PCP, though, that's fine. If they go for an MRI, it's fine. If they go for a "million dollar workup," it's fine. The specialists will establish the needed efficiencies and make the appropriate decisions, at their level. That is not the job of primary care doctors. There should be nothing in what the HMO does that would force primary care physicians out of the traditional family doctor role. No bureaucracy. And no rationing functions. Let other HMOs alienate their PCPs. The overriding goal with this move is that there be a clear and unmistakable differentiation between the flanking HMO and all of the other HMOs with respect to the mythic properties of the doctor/patient relationship.[20]

❑ **Move # 2:** *Establish staff model multispecialty ambulatory care campuses.* These campuses should cover the full continuum of specialty services and be positioned as "one-day health and hospital centers." Each specialty should be managed as a separate business unit and each business unit structured according to a well-defined division of labor. Physicians should all be top-flight specialists. Physicians, nurses, and other technical support staff should all fit into a well-defined division of labor. Staff training should be ongoing, emphasizing both "high-tech" and "high-touch" patient care. And patient visits, whether referred by PCPs or self-referred, should be triaged through specialty-specific production functions. The production functions will enable all cases—from the most trivial to the most complex—to be treated cost-effectively. Move # 2 has four goals: 1) deliver the very best specialty care possible; 2) ensure the clinical efficiency and productive value of each professional's input across the patient care process; 3) build a brand identity associated with absolutely superior specialty medicine; and 4) capture additional fee-for-service patient volume.

---

[20]Many of these points are borne out by current HMO experience. For example, in the August 1992 *Consumer Reports* special series on "Healthcare in Crisis," the lead article stated the following. On broad panels: "Choice, however, is a key to member happiness. 'One of our strong points is a large panel of doctors—6,000,' says Allan Greenberg, chief executive officer of Pilgrim Healthcare, one of the top-rated HMOs in the Ratings. About three-quarters of our readers in Pilgrim's plan were highly satisfied with their doctor" (521). On PCPs not being capitated: "We found a significant relationship between member satisfaction and the way primary care doctors in the HMOs were paid. The HMOs at the top of our Ratings all paid doctors fees for their services" (523). And on the gatekeeper role: "Physicians Health Plan of Minnesota, now called Medica Choice, received the highest rating for member satisfaction with specialists. That isn't surprising, since that group's members can go to any specialist any time without obtaining a referral from a primary care physician" (523).

❑ **Move # 3:** *Establish exclusive channeling relationships with premier hospitals based on capitation and case rate arrangements.* With move # 3, the flanking HMO 1) channels inpatient cases exclusively to the leading hospitals and medical centers in the region; and 2) uses only risk arrangements to compensate said institutions. In exchange for exclusivity, these institutions are either fully capitated or paid all-inclusive case rates. This move allows the flanking HMO to shift the risk for the more costly and acute cases to those facilities most adept at handling them. It also reinforces its reputation as *the* HMO that makes the very best specialty care available to its members.

The three moves outlined above represent a three-pronged risk management strategy:

1. Use primary care to increase enrollment and revenues. Since primary care is not where the major expenses are, it is not where the major savings and efficiencies should be. If total primary care expenditures are at or even a fraction below breakeven, but market share increases significantly, then move # 1 did its job.

2. Use the staff model campuses to enhance the efficiency and coordination of specialty care, plus carve out of the hospital's secondary product those cases that can be treated just as effectively on the ambulatory campuses. A little-known fact outside the HMO industry is that HMOs routinely budget fixed percentages of total premium to broad service categories such as specialists and hospital care. Given internal budgeting at the industry average, move # 2 becomes successful if the staff model campuses provide specialty services better and cheaper than competitors, and if they capture a portion of the operating margin from total premium competitors implicitly allocate to hospitals.

3. Use selected hospitals with the best reputation to take the full risk for all inpatient hospital care. HMOs have already made significant gains in reducing inpatient days. At this point, what is important in the healthcare system is for hospitals themselves to provide inpatient services more cost-effectively. The best way to do that is for hospitals to know they have exclusivity for either all hospital care (capitation) or specific cases (case rates). With exclusivity, they have a budget, and with a budget they have the pre-

dictability needed to reengineer their organization and operations for greater clinical efficiency—the same predictability HMOs strive for through the capitation process. The problem with most current participating relationships, however, is that they don't give hospitals predictability. Move # 3 becomes successful when the flanking HMO truly shifts the risk for inpatient cases to selected premier hospitals and those hospitals are in a position to build ongoing efficiencies across the spectrum of inpatient care.

Assuming industry dynamics run true to form, the flanking HMO should prevail in the HMO marketing wars on three counts: First, creating a tangible differentiation in the primary care doctor/patient relationship; second, building market recognition for big time, institutional capabilities in specialty and hospital care; and third, having a superior economic model.

The superior economic model relates to a comment an actuary made to me a long time ago about health insurance. He said health insurance was ultimately about different pots of money—a point not unlike the one Ries and Trout make about companies with different market positions requiring different strategies. In the case of our flanking HMO, management determined that strategy for the primary care pot should focus on physician and patient satisfaction—saving a penny or two on the dime of primary care in every premium dollar is simply not worth it.

With specialty care, however, the pot is much larger. Here, management in the flanking HMO determined that cost savings is crucial because it applies to a pot perhaps seven times greater than primary care. That is, rather than the dime of every premium dollar allocated to primary care, specialty and hospital care represents at least $.70.[21] Under these circumstances, strategy

---

[21]The $.70 is a per-member per-month (pmpm) estimate for a commercial (under 65) population. It reflects conversations with individuals working in the HMO industry nationally. It consists of approximately $.40 pmpm for specialists and ancillary services and approximately $.30 pmpm for hospitals. It should be emphasized that I am referring to a *single* dollar standard. Typically, for every $100 an HMO receives in premium, primary care represents about $10 pmpm, specialty care and ancillaries about $40 pmpm, and hospital care about $30 pmpm. The remaining $20 is associated with one or another component of administration, operating margin, and statutory reserves. Clearly, these numbers vary somewhat by region and type of HMO. They also depend on how much ancillary and routine specialty work have been shifted to the PCP's area of responsibility and included in their capitation or pmpm payments.

called for establishing greater efficiency on the staff model campuses compared to the discount fee-for-service relationships of competitors. This efficiency, in turn, yields a substantial difference in operating margins. The gains our flanking HMO realizes from its increased margins can then be reinvested to achieve still greater efficiencies as well as lower prices, improved quality, and enhanced service—something the other HMOs cannot do. The cumulative impact of these developments should help our flanking HMO establish a competitive advantage in the marketplace. Insofar as others respond by changing their basic approach to either PCPs or specialists, capitation or discount fee-for-service, *their* battlefield has been shifted. This doesn't mean the HMO wars in that market are over. For now, though, it means the flanking HMO controls the high ground.

Whether competitors genuinely improve themselves and progress in innovative ways or whether they fall into a cycle of mediocrity may well depend on the rules of strategy they choose to adopt. Such rules are a prominent theme in Bruce Henderson's work on corporate strategy, and it is to Henderson that we now turn.

CHAPTER 4

The Rules of Strategy

Machiavelli is generally recognized as the founder of modern political science. In *The Prince*, he formulated a series of maxims the prince needed to follow in order to remain in power. Bruce Henderson, founder of The Boston Consulting Group, writes in a similar vein but from the standpoint of the corporate strategist. In *Henderson on Corporate Strategy*, the author makes a "science" of marketplace relationships much like Machiavelli made a science of political relationships.[1] For Henderson, this is accomplished by showing the predictable impact that different relationships in the marketplace have on competitors and how these relationships require businesses to adopt specific strategies if they are to remain successful.

Towards the end of his book, Henderson writes, "It is obvious that if experience were the only teacher, then we would on average become as competent as our parents only if our life expectancy exceeded theirs. Significant pro-

---

1 Bruce D. Henderson. *Henderson on Corporate Strategy* (New York and Scarborough, Ontario: Mentor Book, New American Library, 1982).

gress in each generation requires a more efficient teacher than experience" (191). The great merit of *Henderson on Corporate Strategy* is that in his hands strategic thinking emerges as an "efficient teacher."

STRATEGIC THINKING AS RENEWAL

For a variety of reasons, change is a basic element in business. World markets change. Local markets change. Technology changes. Competitors change. Even the accepted wisdom changes. Since business conditions are always changing, Henderson states, the "extension of past strategy is essentially a negative course. No matter how well chosen it may be, the fact remains that sooner or later it will become inappropriate" (36).

While change is fundamental to business, Henderson is keenly aware that most organizations have a built-in resistance to change. When companies hit hard times and need new strategies the most, strategy is usually subordinated to operations. Under these circumstances, strategic thinking gains currency only after there has been a change in competitive conditions. Conversely, when companies are successful, there is an overvaluation of established practices, and change becomes taboo. Because "all the forces of corporate culture are set against change," senior management's challenge is to use strategic thinking not just when the need is obvious, but before it is obvious (55). Executives who wait until after problems or opportunities become self-evident may manage, but they won't lead.

According to Henderson, strategic thinking should be an iterative process. That means setting the future course and ensuring that the business stays on course, as well as knowing when to change and what the new change should be. Inhibiting this process, however, is what Henderson calls the "framework of precedent" (36). Since even the most important decisions are made within a framework of precedent, senior management has to continually guard against the past dictating the future.

Henderson is not the first to emphasize the CEO's role in this regard. He does, though, make an important distinction that bears emphasis: "Whereas operating responsibilities can be delegated, strategic planning cannot. Operations can be managed by means of established procedures and controls, but strategic planning requires that all decisions be treated as exceptions" (37). The authority to decide which established practices are functional and which are not—when precedent should be sustained and when it should not—has to flow from the chief executive.

In addition to linking strategic with critical thinking, Henderson makes the point that assumptions, issues, and facts need to be made explicit before they can be explored. "The very lack of explicitness about past and current strategy and the reasons for its success can be an obstacle to accepting the need for change" (36). This point is entirely in keeping with the concept of critique discussed earlier with Tregoe and Zimmerman. For Henderson, the way to make matters explicit is by asking a series of questions in what he calls a "strategy review":[2]

- ❏ What are the products and markets in which we choose to compete?

- ❏ Why has the company succeeded or not succeeded against the competition?

- ❏ Is there a consistent pattern in how the current strategy unfolded?

- ❏ What critical factors were assumed when the strategy was formulated?

- ❏ Have these factors been significantly affected by changes in the marketplace?

- ❏ What should we now be doing differently or better than our competitors?

- ❏ What priorities dictated past resource allocation, and what priorities does the future dictate?

The strategy review does not set strategy so much as it continually reviews the key assumptions underlying strategy. While strategy should not be changed often, the strategy review suggests when strategy should change or, equally important, when the organization should change to support the current strategy. If strategic thinking is to successfully guide a business into the future, it must also be critical, and critical thinking begins with the strategy review.

---

2 These questions are adapted from Henderson, 36 and 41.

RULES FOR RESTRUCTURING THE COMPETITIVE EQUILIBRIUM

As the Ries and Trout chapter demonstrated, military logic has a prominent place in business strategy. Henderson argues, however, that military logic needs to be expanded to include the idea that "business is a continuing process, not just a battle, campaign or even a war to be won and finished" (3). In addition to identifying ways to concentrate one's strengths against a competitor's weaknesses, strategy should view a business and its competitors as a competitive system in equilibrium. "Any really useful strategy must include a means of upsetting the competitive equilibrium and reestablishing it again on a more favorable basis" (3). The perspective should be a dynamic one involving sequence, timing, and competitor reaction—all with the intent of restructuring one's position in the marketplace so it yields a competitive advantage for the long term.

Henderson's comments on sequencing differ from Ohmae's. For Ohmae, sequencing means "sequencing functional competence," reflecting an evolutionary view. For Henderson, sequencing refers to "stages of a business cycle," reflecting more of an economist's view. According to Henderson, it is not only important to invest during growth periods, it may also be important to invest in periods "following high inflation, recession and (even a) liquidity squeeze. . . ." (12). Since these are periods that naturally deter investment, it is the strategist's responsibility to determine when, where, and in what form investment would be most advantageous. Unless you believe that your industry will be forever stuck in the business cycle, Henderson argues, "It should be obvious that investing in capacity before it is needed will be handsomely rewarded" (12). By "capacity," he does not mean the "same old capacity." He means some kind of capacity, whether it be new, different, or the same, just so long as it exploits long-term growth opportunities and competitor weaknesses.

Henderson puts forth a series of rules for the strategist that expand on this last point:[3]

---

[3] Henderson, 13–15. These rules are culled from Henderson's narrative. I have called them "rules." He did not.

- "You must directly or indirectly induce your competitors to refrain from investment in those areas which you find the most attractive for investment."
- "Concentrate your strengths against your competitor's relative weakness" and never attack a stronger, "well-entrenched competitor without first eliminating his ability or willingness to respond in kind."
- "Choose the most vulnerable market segments."
- "Choose products or markets which require response rates beyond a competitor's ability."
- "Choose products or markets which require capital that a competitor is unwilling to commit."
- "Exploit managerial differences in style, method or system, such as overhead rate, distribution channels, market image or flexibility."
- "Appear to be unworthy of attention . . . appear to be unbeatable . . . avoid attention . . . redirect attention . . . appear to be irrational."

Henderson's rule of irrationality follows from the observation that predictability in the marketplace extends beyond the calculus of economic relationships to individuals making decisions about those relationships. With the rule of irrationality, Henderson no longer parallels Machiavelli, but actually adopts some of Machiavelli's reasoning:

> It is worth emphasizing that your competitor is under the maximum handicap if he acts in a completely rational, objective and logical fashion. For then he will cooperate as long as he thinks he can benefit. In fact, if he is completely logical, he will not forgo the profit of cooperation as long as there is *any* net benefit (29).

In that context, Henderson puts forth an additional series of rules for the strategist: (28–34)

- "You must know as accurately as possible just what your competition has at stake. . . . It is not what you gain or lose, but what he gains or loses that sets the limit on his ability to compromise with you."
- "The less the competition knows about your stakes, the less advantage he has. Without a reference point, he does not even know whether you are being unreasonable."

- ❑ "It is absolutely essential to know the character, attitudes, motives and habitual behavior of a competitor if you wish to have a negotiating advantage."
- ❑ "The more arbitrary your demands are, the better your relative competitive position—provided you do not arouse an emotional reaction."
- ❑ "The less arbitrary you seem, the more arbitrary you can in fact be."
- ❑ "Be sure your rival is fully aware of what he can gain if he cooperates and what it will cost him if he does not."
- ❑ "Avoid any action which will arouse your competitor's emotions, since it is essential that he behaves in a logical, reasonable fashion."
- ❑ "Convince your competitor that you are emotionally dedicated to your position and are completely convinced that it is reasonable."
- ❑ "Victory, if achieved, is more often won in the mind of a competitor than in the economic arena."

RULES CONTINUED—MARKET SHARE AND EXPERIENCE CURVE

In addition to rules derived from human psychology, Henderson derives rules from the marketplace as well. These rules are predicated on costs, market share, and the interrelationship between the two—the experience curve. "If an increase in market share is achieved, it can and should result in a proportionate reduction in cost due to the experience curve effect" (12). Those who have the greatest market share, according to Henderson, should also have the lowest costs because their greater share permits greater experience and, by extension, greater efficiencies. "Relative market share and relative accumulated experience become effectively the same over time" (96).

Since market share is positively correlated with efficiency and lower cost, the competitor with the greatest market share should have the greatest cost advantage. This leads Henderson to propose what he calls the "rules of market share." These rules emphasize the strategic importance of market definition and market boundaries. For the strategist, the practical implications are as follows: (98)

- ❑ "Define the market in a way in which you have the greatest inherent cost advantage."

- ❏ "Incur only the costs which *that sector* is willing to pay for."
- ❏ "Concentrate your efforts on obtaining a leading share in *that sector* with the potential cost advantage that leadership offers."
- ❏ "Redefine the markets in adjacent sectors which share experience and cost with the sector in which you are a leader."

Supplementing Henderson's rules of market share is the "Rule of Three and Four." While presented as an hypothesis, the Rule of Three and Four stipulates that a "stable competitive market never has more than three significant competitors, the largest of which never has more than four times the market share of the smallest" (92). Henderson attributes this rule to two empirical observations: First, "A ratio of 2 to 1 in market share between any two competitors seems to be the equilibrium point at which it is neither practical nor advantageous for either competitor to increase or decrease share;" and second, "Any competitor with less than one quarter the share of the largest competitor cannot be an effective competitor" (92).

Henderson proposes another set of rules that follow from the Rule of Three and Four: (93–98)

- ❏ "If there are a large number of competitors, a shakeout is nearly inevitable in the absence of some external constraint or control on competition."
- ❏ "All competitors wishing to survive will have to grow faster than the market in order even to maintain their relative market shares . . . "
- ❏ "All except the two largest share competitors either will be losers, and eventually eliminated, or will be marginal cash traps reporting profits periodically . . . "
- ❏ "The quicker an investment is cashed out or a market position second only to the leader is gained, then the lower the risk and the higher the probable return on investment."
- ❏ "If the low-cost leader holds the price too high, the shakeout will be postponed, and that firm will lose market share until it is no longer a leader."
- ❏ "A challenger expecting to displace an entrenched leader must do so indirectly, by capturing independent sectors, or be prepared to invest far more than the leader will need to invest to defend itself."

❑ "[I]f you cannot be a leader . . . cash out as soon as practical. Take your write-off. Take your tax loss. Take your cash value. Reinvest in products and markets where you can be a successful leader."

❑ "The basic rule is concentrate where you can be a leader."

According to Henderson, competitors with the largest market share have a basic structural advantage. In a spirit not unlike Ries and Trout, he argues that different circumstances present different strategic implications for the market leaders versus those who follow:

❑ "Early market domination is much more valuable than most companies realize. . . . The basic objective in pricing a new product should be to prevent competitors from gaining experience and market share before the new product has achieved major volume. . . . The lower the initial price set by the first producer, the more rapidly that company builds up volume and a differential cost advantage over succeeding competitors, and the faster the market develops" (166–167).

❑ "If you have the lowest cost at nominal capacity, then it is to your advantage to keep prices down sufficiently at all times to dissuade competition from making additional capacity investments unless, of course, you can raise prices and still stay at nominal capacity. Also, it is to your advantage to invest in added capacity as long as you can do so and maintain your cost advantage" (154).

❑ "If your fixed costs are higher but your operating costs are lower than your competitors, then you are more sensitive to changes in operating rate. It is to your advantage to accept any kind of short-term price depression which provides a high operating rate" (155).

❑ "The corporate strategist with the new low-cost facility must persuade competitors that he can and will depress prices indefinitely . . . to the point that the new facility is operating at average industry capacity" (155).

❑ "The strategist who has higher cost facilities but is in possession of the market must convince competitors that high prices for the industry are to everyone's advantage. . . . He may also find it necessary to convince competitors that it will be too costly to wrest his existing market share by price action" (155).

❑ "The perfect strategy for the low-cost producer is one which persuades others to permit him to obtain maximum use of capacity with minimum price depression. . . . The perfect strategy for the high-cost producer is one which persuades others that market shares cannot be shifted except over long periods of time and, therefore, that the highest practical industry prices are to everyone's advantage" (156).

❑ "Paradoxically, it is often the strongest and lowest cost producer which leads the way in establishing higher prices, even though the company itself may be operating below optimum capacity. When this happens, it must be considered a strategic victory for the higher cost producer in the market" (156).

❑ "There are two principal reasons for a shift in market share between competitors. The more common is a lack of capacity. The other is a willingness to lose share to maintain price" (160).

❑ "It is against all logic for high-cost competitors to displace low-cost competitors. But they often do. It seems unreasonable for high-cost competitors to sell at lower prices, grow faster and use more debt than low-cost competition. But they often do. If they did not, then the original leader would never be displaced. Successful business strategy requires that the lowest cost competitor be persuaded indirectly to give up its market share, cost leadership and profitability. This obvious loss to the leader may result from competitors' superior strategy. More often it is a misperception of his own best interests" (108).

HENDERSON, HEALTHCARE AND MANAGED COMPETITION

At first glance, it might appear that Henderson's rules are not entirely applicable to healthcare because the system does not engender price competition. Price, for example, may be a factor influencing patient demand, but since health insurance makes patients less price sensitive, quality and reputation are often more important factors. In addition, the nature of demand in healthcare is unique. Once patients go to physicians, it is not the patient, but the physician who makes the demand decisions. This "supply-induced demand," combined with patients' lack of price sensitivity, undermines the market discipline Henderson's rules assume.

While many aspects of the healthcare system lack price sensitivity, the lack of price sensitivity does not make Henderson's rules any less relevant to healthcare. At most, questions can be raised about two components of his argument: 1) the Rule of Three and Four; and 2) the relationship between cost, market share, and experience.

Regarding the Rule of Three and Four, it should be kept in mind that this is a frame of reference, not a law of physics. If the market share of the top two competitors among insurance companies, hospitals, or even physicians is not two to one, and if the relative market shares of the next two competitors does not conform to some fixed proportion, this does not invalidate the rule. In the medical marketplace, like any marketplace, the two top competitors are likely to enjoy long-term success and competitive advantages while lesser competitors are likely to experience limited success and be at a disadvantage. This picture will continue to apply until circumstances change and market leaders fail to adapt, or until smaller competitors pursue strategies that effectively displace the market leaders.

The relationship between cost, market share, and experience should be considered in two parts: 1) cost/market share and 2) market share/experience. Historically, lower cost has not necessarily increased market share for hospitals and physicians. On the other hand, it is generally recognized that increased market share has increased their experience—that is, stimulated greater efficiencies, economies, and quality. In the clinical context, for example, the more procedures a surgical team performs, the more efficient its use of the operating room and the better the expected outcome. The same principle applies to an individual surgeon, specialist, or generalist whose reputation attracts certain kinds of cases, which in turn enables the practitioner to further refine his or her own clinical expertise. This is the main assumption underlying the move to centers of excellence in healthcare today.

Having said that, it must be emphasized that while lower cost has not correlated with increased market share in the past, current attempts to control healthcare inflation through "managed competition" suggest that it will in the future. Managed competition is a policy embraced by both government and private employers to achieve market reforms by further stimulating managed care developments of the 1980s. Managed care includes 1) HMOs and PPOs as an alternative to traditional health insurance, 2) incorporation of preauthorization procedures into traditional health insurance, 3) reliance on primary care physicians (PCPs) as "gatekeepers" to coordinate individuals' use of medical services and regulate access to specialists, and 4) standardized clinical protocols plus other utilization management techniques to facilitate cost-effective practice patterns among physicians.

The assumption behind managed competition is that people will switch from health coverage tied to independent providers in an open-ended fee-for-service environment to health coverage tied to providers in managed care systems. These systems, such as HMOs, PPOs, and hybrid point-of-service plans, are designed to regulate the cost of internal patient transactions. What is significant about managed competition is that it represents a widely held view that endorses *financial incentives* as the means for getting people to switch from traditional health insurance to managed care systems.[4] While the specifics of these incentives may change, the goal to increase price sensitivity among individuals in selecting their mode of health coverage will not. With increased price sensitivity, the medical marketplace is expected to become competitive in three fundamental ways:

❑ As people experience the difference in premium and out-of-pocket costs between traditional health insurance and managed care systems, they will eventually become price sensitive.

❑ As people become price sensitive, managed care systems will become price competitive.

❑ As managed care systems become price competitive, traditional health insurers will themselves be forced to convert to managed care in order to compete on price.

Under managed competition, therefore, industry dynamics associated with a more price-competitive marketplace will begin to shape *organizational be-*

---

4 The most straightforward financial incentive is for employers to limit their premium contributions to employee health benefits so that employees will be completely responsible for anything above a certain dollar amount. An extension of this approach is to tax employee health benefits above a certain amount and to limit the premium employers can deduct as a business expense. Under current law, the health benefit that workers receive from their employers is not considered taxable income, and employers are allowed to deduct the entire cost of health insurance as a business expense. By placing limits on both employees' tax free health benefit as well as the amount of premium employers can deduct and pegging those limits to the premium of an average-priced managed care plan, the assumption is that employers and employees will become far more price sensitive with respect to health coverage. This price sensitivity, in turn, will make individual managed care systems (HMOs, PPOs, etc.) more price competitive.

havior throughout healthcare delivery. From the standpoint of Henderson's rules, this suggests that where lower cost and increased market share may not have been entirely applicable to health insurance, hospitals, or physicians in the past, they will be increasingly applicable in the future.

MANAGED COMPETITION AND COMMODIFICATION

There is an undeniable commodity quality in Henderson's reasoning that did not exist in healthcare until recently. Such factors as physicians' "professional authority," the patient's "sick role," and the "mystique" of medical science all served to prevent commodity considerations from entering into healthcare. In addition, the marriage of medical science and the medical profession legitimized the profession's special authority. Since both "doctoring" and "science" were supposed to be objective and detached, an ideology existed throughout most of the 20th century that nothing should get in between the doctor and patient. This ideology insulated physicians' clinical decision making from Adam Smith's "hidden hand." It also prevented commodity considerations from entering into the imagery people associated with medicine. The ideology was reinforced by the prerogatives the government granted the medical profession to license and regulate itself. Most importantly, though, it was institutionalized by the *separation of health insurance from healthcare delivery.*

That separation defined the nature of health insurance in the United States. It was a precondition for the medical profession's support of private health insurance after 1945; it formed the foundation of employer-based coverage which expanded dramatically in the late 1940s and 1950s; and it framed the basic approach of Medicare and Medicaid after 1965. In addition, the separation of health insurance from healthcare delivery conditioned healthcare industry behavior in two significant ways:

❏ First, it preserved the cottage industry structure of the medical profession by preventing the imperatives of corporate organization from being imposed on physicians. Regardless of how high-tech medicine became, the medical profession remained, in a sense, preindustrial—that is, physicians continued to "ply their trade" as independent artisans.

❏ Second, it established the principle of indemnification in traditional health insurance. Indemnification gave patients free reign to choose their providers and then compensated them for most of the full price providers charged. It also enabled patients to think in terms of benefit alone, as opposed to cost and benefit, when paying for medical care. As a result, healthcare services retained their "qualitative" nature, rather than taking on industrial qualities and becoming more "quantitative" in nature.

The combined impact of these two factors prevented patients, providers, and even payors from relating to healthcare in commodity terms. With managed competition, however, each of these factors is negated:

❑ First, health coverage is formally linked to managed care systems, reducing the earlier separation of health insurance from healthcare delivery. These systems now bring physicians (as well as hospitals and other providers) into a corporate framework so clinical activity can be made to conform to organizational requirements.

❑ Second, health insurance is recast from indemnifying medical services to subsidizing the selection of managed care systems that deliver medical services. People, in other words, are expected to choose managed care systems like they would cars or computers. For their part, physicians in these systems are expected to make clinical decisions like any manager who has to consider the cost of inputs.

Managed competition's transformation of healthcare into a commodity represents a paradigm shift in healthcare delivery. For better or worse, the more this process proceeds, the more applicable Henderson's rules of strategy become.

RISK AND MANAGED COMPETITION

One of the enduring myths about the health insurance industry in the United States is that insurance companies go at risk when they sell health coverage. I would argue the exact opposite has been the case. People go at risk when they buy stocks because if the stock goes down, they lose money. Venture capitalists go at risk because if their investment fails, they lose money. Health insurance companies, however, do not go at risk when they sell policies: If they incur loses, they simply raise premiums. This applies to traditional health insurance as well as managed care health insurance. In theory, then, while the traditional and managed care sides of the industry represent entirely different approaches to offering coverage, in practice they have been more similar than is generally recognized. It is this similarity that makes healthcare ripe for managed competition.

A key structural change underlying managed competition is that price competition among systems of managed care promises to force most of the health insurance industry into going at risk. That is, rather than health insurers having some kind of sinecure relationship to the public that entitles them to cover losses with annual premium increases, like a General Motors, Sears, or IBM, health insurers will have to absorb their losses, restructure their businesses, and develop new programs and services to earn future profits. And they will have to do so while still pricing their products competitively. Whether and how the various industry players under managed competition accept that challenge may ultimately determine if healthcare inflation can be controlled by the marketplace.

In health insurance generally, it should be noted that there are important differences in the industry position of traditional health insurance carriers, PPOs, and HMOs around the approach to risk management and that industry dynamics of managed competition impact these differences in very distinct ways. A standard way of depicting how traditional and managed care insurers differ is along three dimensions of risk management: 1) freedom of choice, 2) utilization management, and 3) approach to reimbursement.[5] These dimensions are displayed in Figure 4–1.

What this figure shows is that as we move from left to right, from traditional health insurance through PPOs to HMOs 1) consumers have less freedom of choice; 2) various forms of utilization review and utilization management are more formally integrated in provider activity; and 3) capitation emerges as a central element along with discount fee-for-service in provider reimbursement. As a result, it is generally assumed that risk management becomes more effective in PPOs compared to traditional insurance and more effective in HMOs compared to PPOs.

What Henderson would argue is that the approach to risk management is the key link between the health insurance industry on the one hand and the all important relationships of cost, market share, and experience on the other. In principle, the more successful the approach to risk management, the lower the costs, the greater the share, and the greater the experience. I

---

5 Fee-for-service, associated with traditional insurance and PPOs, uses deductibles, coinsurance, and co-payments to discipline patient demand. Capitation, associated with HMOs, uses a fixed budget to discipline provider or supply-induced demand.

Figure 4–1.   Dimensions of Risk Management in Health Insurance

| Traditional | Managed Care | | |
	PPOs	POS	HMOs

♦Freedom of
  Choice
♦Indemnity
  Reimbursement
	♦Out-of-Panel
	  Coverage
	♦Discount Fee-for-
	  Service
	♦Some Utilization
	  "Review"
	 _Preauthorization
	 _Retrospective
	  Review
	 _Catastrophic Case
	  Management
			♦No Out-of-Pocket
			  Coverage
			♦Discount Fee-for-
			  Service
			♦Capitalization
			♦Strong Utilization
			  "Management"
			 -Standardized
			  Protocols
			 -PCP Gatekeepers
			 -Preauthorization
			 -Concurrent Review
			 -Retrospective Review
			 -Catastrophic Case
			  Management
			 -Physician Profiling

♦Preauthorization Requirements			

do not believe this principle holds true in the HMO arena, though, because for most HMOs fee-for-service continues to co-exist with capitation. As shown in Figure 4–2, there is almost always fee-for-service reimbursement within HMO delivery systems.

While fee-for-service is discount based and employed as a means of paying providers out of a total budget, it does not replace capitation:

❑ In some cases, fee-for-service operates between payor and provider *directly*, so the orbit inside the HMO delivery system is really no different than a traditional insurance or PPO environment. These direct contract models include classic IPA HMOs and their next generation gatekeeper/PCP counterparts.

❑ In other cases, fee-for-service operates between payor and provider *indirectly*, with the orbit outside the HMO but inside the delivery system with which the HMO contracts. These indirect contract models—often called health plans—are defined by the HMO capitating separate physician-sponsored IPAs, medical groups, and PHOs. Despite the different structural context, gatekeeper/PCPs are prevalent in this second case as well.

The trend in the HMO industry is toward the second case—indirect contract models or health plans. Implicit in these arrangements is the migration

Figure 4–2.   Fee-for-Service Orbits Among HMO Types

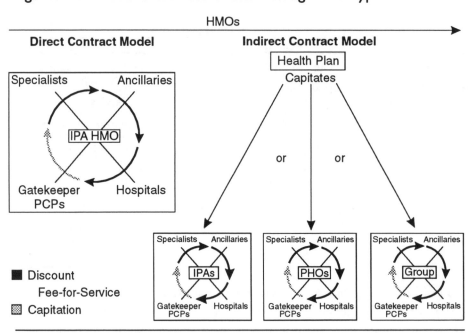

of risk from the HMO to the provider entity. Whether an HMO contracts with an IPA, a PHO, or a medical group is largely dependent on local circumstances. For physicians, hospitals, and other service vendors, such entities represent *distribution systems* for access to patients. If providers are not part of the winning distribution system in the local market, they stand a good chance of losing much of their HMO patient base. Clearly, from a competitive standpoint, battles will be fought over which distribution system is to be used by HMOs. Not so clear from an industry standpoint, however, are the performance implications associated with the commingling of fee-for-service and capitation in HMOs.

What Henderson's rules suggest is that HMOs' continued reliance on fee-for-service prevents the formation of *production capabilities* that support the two primary goals of capitation: 1) offering a comprehensive benefit comparable to traditional health insurance but at a lower price, and 2) lowering the actual cost of producing healthcare services. While the perverse incentive of fee-for-service in HMOs is diminished, due primarily to aggressive utilization management, fee-for-service remains inimical to the cost advantage capitation is expected to achieve.

For Henderson, a central factor in strategic thinking is the capability of one player to establish a cost advantage over others. *Direct your capability to the market that gives you the greatest inherent cost advantage. Wield your capability in ways the market is willing to pay for. Refine your capability to fully exploit your cost advantage. Expand your capability to other markets that share the cost and experience curve of the capability that either made you a leader or can make you a leader. The basic rule is concentrate on your capabilities.*[6]

In health insurance, the approach to risk management goes to the heart of what Henderson calls "capability." The approach has to be internally consistent with the product the health insurer is expected to deliver. To the extent that the approach to risk management is compromised, conditions favoring a cost advantage are also compromised. More likely than not, the product will suffer as well.

Applying Henderson's thinking to managed competition, the inference I draw from his rules is that capitation and fee-for-service presuppose different managed care products and that these products are tied to different kinds of delivery systems. To catch a glimpse at the future of healthcare under managed competition, look to the *structural relationship* between the products and performance of delivery systems under capitation versus fee-for-service. Putting it baldly, I would argue the following:

Managed Care Products:

1. Those who want a comprehensive and coordinated healthcare product and do not want to pay more than a token amount each time they visit a provider will want managed care systems organized around capitation. Under managed competition, the capitated systems producing this product the best will be staff or salaried group model HMOs—a Harvard Community Health Plan, a Geisinger Health Plan, a Kaiser Permanente, or a Group Health of Puget Sound.

2. Those who want a product with freedom of choice, multiple options in benefit packages, and the flexibility to annually change their out-of-pocket liabilities, will want managed care systems predicated on fee-for-service. Under managed competition, the

---

6 Adapted from the "rules" listed earlier in this chapter.

fee-for-service systems producing this product the best will be point-of-service plans and PPOs that obtain the best discounts with participating providers, have the most attractive provider panels, and marry discounts and provider panels to benefit design options in the most creative ways.

Managed Care Performance:

1. With capitation, the thrust should be towards staff or salaried group model HMOs because they are truly integrated delivery systems with the capacity to recycle gains made from increased experience back into a single organization responsible for the production of health services. The capacity to recycle experience in this way puts such systems in a position to achieve clinical efficiencies that yield, arguably, the most crucial source of cost advantage.[7]

2. With fee-for-service, the thrust should be towards arrangements that make healthcare services available for people to *buy*. Managed care systems positioned as arrangements can achieve their cost advantage by careful actuarial pricing and prudent benefit designs, combined with strong vendor agreements to allow for more efficient purchasing.

---

[7] Many hospital systems, hospitals, and large medical groups have either developed or are planning to develop "integrated delivery systems" as their principle strategy for approaching managed care in the marketplace. I believe this trend is inherently flawed because such systems are usually umbrella organizations only. The label "integrated" is due to their containing a full menu of provider organizations under one roof: medical groups, IPAs, PHOs, hospitals, individual participating physicians, and ancillary service agreements. While there may well be staff or salaried group components, the inference that integration exists is not only wrong but deceptive since integration does not take place at the level where health services are literally produced. Currently, "integrated delivery systems" are really more like a diversified corporation with a number of related businesses that are capable of co-venturing for contracting purposes. As a general rule, I would argue that where the delivery system is not a staff model or salaried group, it is not truly integrated. The exception to this rule, which will be discussed at length in Chapter 6, is if the infrastructure supporting nonstaff or nonsalaried group arrangements (i.e., PPOs, POS plans, or IPAs) is thoroughly "informationalized." A comprehensive on-line, real-time management information system that completely links clinical and administrative components for all of the participating providers can transform nonstaff or nonsalaried arrangements into integrated delivery systems.

A fundamental difference between managed care systems predicated on capitation versus fee-for-service is that *staff and salaried group model HMOs can feed back experience and knowledge to a single organization to improve production capability and efficiency at the level of medical practice; whereas, arrangements cannot.* Insofar as HMOs continue to rely on fee-for-service by either directly contracting with providers or indirectly contracting with separate provider organizations that distribute their capitation through fee-for-service, they elevate purchasing over production and arrangements over functional integration in the day-to-day delivery of health services. This tendency creates all sorts of inconsistencies in the inner workings of "fee-for-service HMOs" and prevents such HMOs from having the capabilities that can yield a sustainable cost advantage.[8]

It is conceivable, of course, that in certain markets fee-for-service HMOs will cost less than staff and salaried group model HMOs. It is also conceivable that patients will feel fee-for-service HMOs provide better quality of care. Following Henderson, though, the explanation rests in the latter's inability to effectively *concentrate on production.*

HENDERSON AND HMO INDUSTRY EVOLUTION

Despite the mergers and consolidation now underway in the HMO sector, managed competition itself is in its developing or growth phase of industry evolution.[9] According to Henderson, the cardinal rule at such times should be to aggressively exploit market-share opportunities. *Early market domination is much more valuable than most companies realize. The basic objective*

---

8 New Jersey Blue Cross and Blue Shield recently came to this conclusion with the adoption of an entirely new strategy for its IPA model HMO. According to the *New York Times*, the Plan is committed to building "a statewide system of private family clinics, putting the company in the business of directly providing healthcare as well as insurance." Quoting from the *Times* further, "Blue Cross officials said they anticipate that the company's own healthcare centers would drive down the overall cost for its managed care system by 15 percent and that they intended to pass along those savings to those subscribers who opted for that plan." Jerry Gray. "Blue Cross Says It Plans Clinics In New Jersey." *New York Times* (May 20, 1994): B1. Aetna, Cigna and PruCare are also beginning to move in this direction through limited physician acquisition/staff model initiatives of their own; see Chris Roush. "Your Doctor's Boss May Be An Insurance Company." *Business Week* (September 19, 1994): 112.

9 This point is discussed at length in Chapter 5.

should be to prevent competitors from gaining experience and market share. The lower the initial price set, the more rapidly the company builds up volume and a differential cost advantage. Successful strategy requires the lowest possible prices.[10]

From Henderson's standpoint, HMOs should do everything possible to lower their costs, but they should lower their costs compared to other HMOs. I mention this because there is a tendency for HMOs to redefine their industry position in order to capture other segments of the market oriented to freedom of choice.[11] Aside from blurring the market's perception of what an HMO is, this orientation pushes HMOs into the trap of competing on multiple fronts—competing for traditional indemnity and PPO business—when they should only compete for HMO business. While out-of-panel or point-of-service options may seem attractive to the market, the intent for HMOs should be to deliver on the cost containment and product potential HMOs are specifically expected to offer. If benefit designs are expanded to include PPO-like options, the HMO delivery system is compromised. Applying Henderson's reasoning, HMOs should stick to being HMOs and continuously improve their capacity to produce a high-quality, comprehensive product at the lowest possible price.

In the last section, I argued that unlike PPOs or POS plans, HMOs *can* feed back experience and learning curve to the organization because they are based on capitation. This does not mean they do or that they do so equally. The structure of the HMO determines whether and how effectively this process occurs.

An inherent weakness in fee-for-service HMOs, however, is that physicians still work in their own private practices. What HMO organization exists, exists as *administration* over such activities as claims processing, utilization management, and provider relations—activities designed to impose control over independent physicians. Consequently, any gains fee-for-service HMOs realize from the experience curve impact *bureaucratic functions*, not the pro-

---

[10]Adapted from the "rules" listed earlier in this chapter.

[11]Linda Koco. "Competition Spurs Growth of Point-of-Service HMOs; Point-of-Service HMOs Will Grow Like Corn." *National Underwriter (Life/Health/Financial Services)* 95 (April 29, 1991): 7–9; Linda Koco. "Point-of-Service HMOs Are Growing Rapidly." *National Underwriter (Life/Health/Financial Services)* 95 (June 10, 1991): 15, 17.

duction of medical care per se. In the long run, I do not believe these bureaucratic gains will create significant cost advantages for HMOs.

Staff and salaried group model HMOs, on the other hand, do not have individual physicians spread out in private practices. Physicians operate within an integrated delivery system. Here, gains from increased experience feed back directly to the organization and medical practice. In the long run, I believe these gains have the potential to create significant cost advantages for HMOs. HMOs realizing the greatest cost advantage will be those that are the most successful in bringing clinical, technological, and organizational innovations *into the production process of medical practice*. If Henderson's rules tell us anything, it is that those HMOs should be the HMO market leaders.

It bears emphasizing that the cost advantage market leaders realize should yield still greater market penetration, which in turn should yield greater experience, improved margins, enhanced quality, and the opportunity to reinvest. I say this because staff and salaried group model HMOs have a reputation—deserving or not—of providing lower quality of care. However, the more that successful HMOs gain share and experience, the more they are in a position to reinvest in clinical programs to upgrade quality of care. In Ohmae's terms, the more they can sequence improvement in key functional areas and, like Honda, progress from a low-end "Civic" to a high-end "Acura." To the extent they do not, I suspect in most instances the problem rests with management.

At some point, there may well be no additional market share to capture. Henderson would argue that when this happens, the market leader should not redefine itself by offering out-of-panel coverage or becoming something HMOs are not. Market leaders should continue to invest to maintain their cost differential, improve their capacity, and expand to contiguous markets. While they might also diversify, diversification should either strengthen the core business or be organized as a separate business in order not to confound the HMO itself. Remember, *it is against all logic for a high-cost competitor to displace the low-cost market leader. But they often do. When this happens, it may result from the competitor's superior strategy. More often, though, it results from a misperception of the leader's best interests.*[12]

---

[12]Adapted from the "rules" listed earlier in this chapter.

THE PRODUCT PORTFOLIO

From time to time, it is important for businesses with multiple products to strategically review their product portfolio in light of future corporate commitments. Henderson and The Boston Consulting Group were pioneers in developing the technique called "portfolio analysis" for just that purpose.

Portfolio analysis allows management to evaluate the role different products should play in the context of a company's overall product mix. Through portfolio analysis, companies avoid the pitfall of spreading themselves too thin by investing in all products equally. Rather than diluting the potential of one or another product, portfolio analysis enables management to concentrate resources where growth and profit potential are the greatest. Portfolio analysis also allows management to periodically eliminate products that are floundering and to invest in still-questionable products that show promise.

For Henderson, portfolio analysis revolves around two business variables impacting a third business requirement: growth and market share impacting cash flow.[13] Henderson suggests four rules for categorizing a series of relationships: (168)

- ❑ "Margins and cash are a function of market share. High margins and high market share go together. This . . . is explained by the experience curve effect."

- ❑ "Growth requires cash inputs to finance added assets. The added cash required to hold share is a function of growth rates."

- ❑ "High market share must be earned or bought. Buying market share requires additional investment."

- ❑ "No product market can grow indefinitely. The payoff for growth must come when growth slows, or it will not come at all. The payoff is cash that cannot be reinvested in that product."

Accordingly, a company's products fall into one of four categories: Stars, cash cows, problem children, and dogs.[14] These categories, and various cash flow scenarios, are depicted in Figure 4–3.

---

[13]Other respected approaches to portfolio analysis are described in Appendix B.
[14]This summary is based heavily on Henderson's text, 168–171.

Figure 4–3.   Product Portfolio Matrix

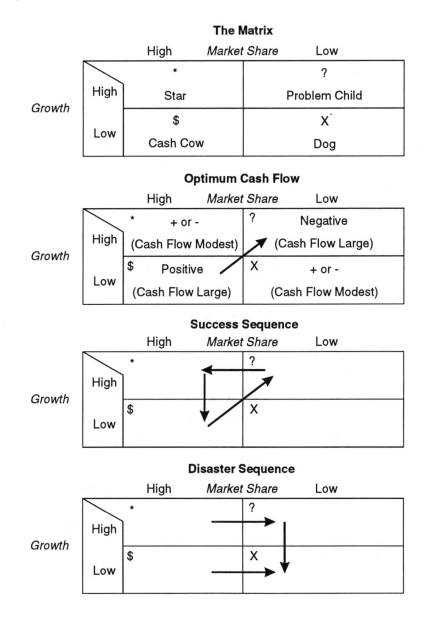

The Matrix

Optimum Cash Flow

Success Sequence

Disaster Sequence

Source: Reprinted from Bruce Henderson, *Henderson on Corporate Strategy* (New York and Scarborough, Ontario: Mentor Book; New American Library, 1982). Used by permission of The Boston Consulting Group, Inc., Boston, Massachusetts.

Cash cows are products with high market share in slow-growth industries. They generate large amounts of cash, amounts that exceed what is required to maintain market share. This excess should not be reinvested in the cash cow because it will only realize a declining rate of return.

Problem children are products that require more cash than they can generate. Their high growth/low market share profile is the issue management must resolve. If such products do not receive additional cash infusions, it is unlikely they will gain market share. But if they do get that infusion, gains in market share are not automatic. The product still needs to compete effectively. Optimally, senior management chooses the right problem child, and the additional investment comes from its cash cow.

Stars have high market share in high-growth industries. They are distinguished not only by profits, but by growing profits. To maintain leadership, stars reinvest from their own revenue, though they may well draw on additional corporate capital. When industry growth slows, stars become cash cows (throwing off cash) for reinvestment elsewhere.

Dogs have low market share in low-growth industries. They may show occasional profits, but the dominant pattern is that they consume more resources than they generate. Dogs are a drag on a company's portfolio and should either be sold, spun off, or liquidated. They represent failures.

As the earlier discussion on Henderson would suggest, "The value of a product is completely dependent upon obtaining a leading share of its market before the growth slows" (169). After growth slows, profits drop. Eventually, all products become either cash cows or dogs.

A NOTE ON PORTFOLIO ANALYSIS IN HEALTHCARE

Portfolio analysis is more applicable in institutional settings than individual settings. It is also more applicable in healthcare situations where the relationships of cost, market share, and experience hold true and less applicable where they do not. A single internist practicing in a private office will have little use for portfolio analysis because he or she really offers no one, basic product. A multispecialty group, on the other hand, will have greater use for portfolio analysis because the complement of physicians under one roof may have specialty or subspecialty capabilities that can be leveraged in a variety of ways.

Obviously, hospitals support multiple clinical services and are in a position to define cash cows and problem children, stars and dogs. Whether they are free to act on these definitions is another matter. Hospitals may well be obligated to maintain certain services even if they do not make good business sense because to do otherwise would violate their community responsibility. How they cross-subsidize those services is the issue.

Extending Henderson's reasoning, one role for local philanthropy in hospitals might well be to support programs and services that are needed in the community but are considered dogs or problem children. Philosophically, this could help resolve some of the anomalies associated with business in medicine. It could, for instance, free the profitable components of hospital activity from supporting the nonprofitable components, enabling the former to be disciplined by the marketplace, while the latter is sustained by philanthropy. Indeed, it could be argued that when philanthropy cross-subsidizes profitable hospital services, those services lose their competitive edge, just as those same services lose their competitive edge when they subsidize unprofitable services by throwing off capital needed for their own future growth.

Health insurance companies are in a less-sensitive situation relative to the community. Whether they apply portfolio analysis, and how they do so, is more a function of corporate politics than anything else. Again, going back to a point made earlier in this chapter, "All the forces of corporate culture are set against change" (55). Since portfolio analysis by its very nature creates change, the conditions under which it operates are rarely hospitable. When portfolio analysis is used by health insurers to reevaluate future direction, any number of areas in the insurer's organization could be greatly affected. Suffice it to say, it is then that the need for leadership is greatest.

CHAPTER 5

Industry Structure and Strategy

Michael Porter's two books, *Competitive Strategy* and *Competitive Advantage*, are both enormously comprehensive texts that analyze various aspects of business strategy.[1] *Competitive Strategy* focuses on how industry structure and market forces affect the conditions that need to be understood in formulating strategy. *Competitive Advantage* focuses on how business strategy can create and sustain market leadership. The two texts represent a single line of thought, with the second building on the first. In *Competitive Strategy*, Porter elaborates on the two broad forms of competitive advantage: Cost leadership and differentiation. In *Competitive Advantage*, he elaborates on the role a firm's "value chain" plays in business strategy. The value chain is a series of functional activities all firms engage in to conduct business.

---

[1] Michael E. Porter. *Competitive Strategy: Techniques for Analyzing Industries and Competitors* (New York: The Free Press, 1980); and Michael Porter. *Competitive Advantage: Creating and Sustaining Superior Performance* (New York: The Free Press, 1985).

According to Porter, a firm's value chain is the ultimate basis for succeeding through either low cost or differentiation.

Like good therapy, strategically oriented businesses are consistently governed by analytic detail they are never fully conscious of. It is this unconscious knowledge that makes for successful businesses. Such awareness doesn't just come together naturally, though. It takes work. Porter's great contribution is that his two volumes on strategy serve as an invaluable resource for businesses to do *that* work.

INDUSTRY STRUCTURE AND COMPETITIVE FORCES

Industry structure is the sum total of competitive forces and relationships that shape the overall context of an industry.[2] It is industry structure that conditions the conduct of business and an industry's profit potential. Industry structure, for Porter, revolves around five basic competitive forces: 1) threat of new market entrants, 2) threat of substitute products, 3) bargaining power of buyers, 4) bargaining power of suppliers, and 5) intensity of rivalry among existing firms.

1.   The greater the threat of new market entrants, the greater the competition expected in an industry, and the greater the downward pressure on prices. The threat of new market entrants depends primarily on entry barriers:

   ❑ Economies of scale.[3]

   ❑ Product differentiation.[4]

   ❑ Capital requirements.

   ❑ Switching costs.

   ❑ Access to distribution channels.

---

2 This section summarizes Porter, 1980, 3–33.

3 Scale requirements can relate to any business function. In addition, they change as technology changes.

4 Differentiation can result from previous advertising, strong or unique customer service, product differences, or having been first in an industry.

□ Disadvantages independent of scale.[5]

□ Government policies.[6]

□ Expected retaliation.[7]

2. Substitution is a second competitive force that shapes industry profitability. Whether and to what degree the threat of substitute products exists depends on at least four factors:

□ The price-performance alternative offered by substitutes.

□ Technological developments.

□ Switching costs.

□ An industry's collective potential to preempt substitution.

3. Buyers can affect industry profitability through demands for lower prices, more services, specific product or service requirements, and better quality. The bargaining power of buyers is stronger when any of the following exist:

□ Buyer is a major or *the* major purchaser of a seller.

□ Purchased goods or services represent a significant fraction of the buyer's costs.

□ Purchased goods are standard or undifferentiated.

□ Buyer confronts relatively small switching costs.

□ Buyer is price sensitive because of low profit margins.

□ Buyer is a credible threat for backward integration.

□ The product being bought is either unimportant or vulnerable to substitution.

□ Buyer has full information.

---

[5] This occurs when established firms possess advantages that have nothing to do with, and cannot be overcome by, size or economies of scale (e.g., proprietary technology, favorable locations, or government subsidies).

[6] For example, licensing, regulation, and performance standards.

[7] Signs of potentially significant retaliation include a history of retaliation against new entrants, existing firms having the strength to retaliate, one or more firms having a strong commitment to preserve the current competitor mix, and slow industry growth.

4. Suppliers affect industry profitability by raising prices or changing the quality of goods and services supplied. The bargaining power of suppliers is increased when:

   ❑ There are few suppliers and suppliers are more concentrated than buyers.

   ❑ Suppliers have no threat of substitute products.

   ❑ The industry is not an important customer of suppliers.

   ❑ The supplier's product or service is important to the buyer's business.

   ❑ The supplier's products are well differentiated and buyers face high switching costs.

   ❑ The supplier is a credible threat for forward integration.

5. The intensity of rivalry among existing competitors is perhaps the most classic competitive force in an industry. While rivalry depends on competitors themselves, it also depends on how other competitive forces play out. Competitive rivalry, then, results from a number of different factors:

   ❑ Numerous or equally balanced competitors.

   ❑ Slow industry growth.

   ❑ High fixed or storage costs, which can lead to rapid price cutting when excess capacity is present.

   ❑ Capacity augmented in large increments, which can lead to disruption in stable supply/demand relationships.

   ❑ Lack of differentiation.

   ❑ Minimal switching costs.

   ❑ Diverse competitors.

   ❑ Competitors placing strategic value in the same area.

   ❑ High exit barriers.

Figure 5–1 summarizes the five competitive forces affecting industry structure and profitability.

Figure 5–1.   Elements of Industry Structure

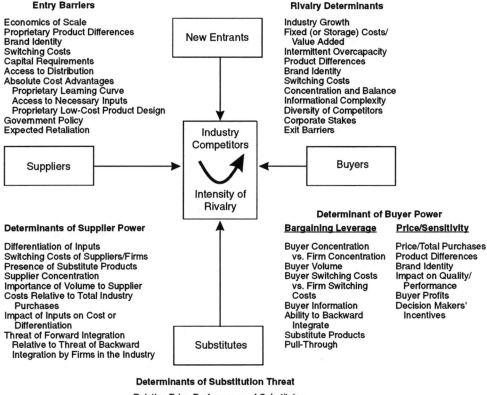

Entry Barriers

Economics of Scale
Proprietary Product Differences
Brand Identity
Switching Costs
Capital Requirements
Access to Distribution
Absolute Cost Advantages
  Proprietary Learning Curve
  Access to Necessary Inputs
  Proprietary Low-Cost Product Design
Government Policy
Expected Retaliation

Rivalry Determinants

Industry Growth
Fixed (or Storage) Costs/
  Value Added
Intermittent Overcapacity
Product Differences
Brand Identity
Switching Costs
Concentration and Balance
Informational Complexity
Diversity of Competitors
Corporate Stakes
Exit Barriers

New Entrants

Industry Competitors

Suppliers → ← Buyers

Intensity of Rivalry

Determinants of Supplier Power

Differentiation of Inputs
Switching Costs of Suppliers/Firms
Presence of Substitute Products
Supplier Concentration
Importance of Volume to Supplier
Costs Relative to Total Industry
  Purchases
Impact of Inputs on Cost or
  Differentiation
Threat of Forward Integration
  Relative to Threat of Backward
  Integration by Firms in the Industry

Determinant of Buyer Power

Bargaining Leverage

Buyer Concentration
  vs. Firm Concentration
Buyer Volume
Buyer Switching Costs
  vs. Firm Switching
  Costs
Buyer Information
Ability to Backward
  Integrate
Substitute Products
Pull-Through

Price/Sensitivity

Price/Total Purchases
Product Differences
Brand Identity
Impact on Quality/
  Performance
Buyer Profits
Decision Makers'
  Incentives

Substitutes

Determinants of Substitution Threat

Relative Price Performance of Substitutes
Switching Costs
Buyer Propensity to Substitute

Source: Reprinted with the permission of The Free Press, a Division of Simon & Schuster from *Competitive Advantage: Creating and Sustaining Superior Performance* by Michael E. Porter. Copyright © 1985 by Michael E. Porter.

GENERIC INDUSTRY STRATEGIES

Strategic thinking involves the search for the most favorable competitive position in an industry. For Porter, two core questions underlie the choice of strategy. In what ways is an industry attractive from the standpoint of long-term profitability? And what are the determinants for competitive advantage? (1985, 1) The last section addressed the first question. This section will begin to address the second.

At the broadest level, there are two kinds of competitive advantage: Cost leadership and differentiation. Each of these represents what Porter calls "generic strategies." A third generic strategy is a subset of the other two. This strategy is focus. The three generic strategies are described below:

❑ **Cost Leadership.** When striving to be the cost leader, cost reduction becomes the major theme running throughout strategy. A low-cost strategy addresses facility; operations; overhead; cost savings from experience; avoiding marginal customers; and being relatively tight-fisted in such areas as R&D, service, sales force, training and development, and advertising. Overall cost leadership "gives the firm a defense against rivalry from competitors because its lower costs mean that it can still earn returns after competitors have competed away their profits through rivalry. A low cost position defends the firm against powerful buyers because buyers can exert power only to drive down prices to the level of the next most efficient competitor. Low cost provides a defense against powerful suppliers by providing more flexibility to cope with input cost increases. The factors that lead to a low cost position . . . also provide substantial entry barriers in terms of scale. . . . Finally, a low cost position . . . places the firm in a favorable position vis-á-vis substitutes. . . . Thus, a low cost position protects the firm against all five competitive forces (1980, 35–36).

❑ **Differentiation.** Strategies based on differentiation seek to establish fundamental differences in a variety of dimensions so that buyers perceive a marked contrast between one firm and its rivals. Firms that successfully differentiate themselves are rewarded for their uniqueness with a premium price. The economics inherent in this generic strategy require that the premium exceed the extra cost incurred in being unique. Differentiation cannot ignore cost issues, therefore, because premium prices will be nullified by inordinately high costs. Firms that differentiate themselves successfully also create a defensible position against the five competitive forces. "Differentiation provides insulation against competitive rivalry because of brand loyalty. . . . The resulting customer loyalty and need for a competitor to overcome uniqueness provide entry barriers. Differentiation yields high margins with which to deal with supplier power, and it clearly mitigates buyer power since buyers lack comparable alternatives and are thereby less price sensitive. Finally, the firm that has differentiated itself to achieve customer loyalty should be better positioned vis-á-vis substitutes than its competitors" (1980, 37–38; 1985, 14).

❑ **Focus.** The last of the three generic strategies is focus. Firms that adopt a focus strategy target narrow market segments rather than the market as a whole. To succeed, they still need to achieve either cost leadership or effective differentiation, but their market is more limited in scale. Through cost focus or differentiation focus, firms seek to exploit differences between what they can do for specific segments versus what their competitors can do. These differences imply that the segments are more poorly served by broad-based competitors than they would be by competitors who served them alone. By directing a firm's capabilities to specific target segments, the focuser seeks a competitive advantage even though it does not possess a competitive advantage in the market overall. One prerequisite for a focus strategy is that the target segments are somehow different than other segments in the market (1985, 15–16; 1980, 38–40).

Not unlike the point made by Tregoe and Zimmerman—that a business should commit to one and only one driving force—Porter emphasizes that a business should commit to one and only one generic strategy. Failing that, firms, in Porter's words, are "stuck in the middle." Such firms lack "the market share, capital investment, and resolve to play the low-cost game, the industrywide differentiation necessary to obviate the need for a low-cost position, or the focus to create differentiation or low cost in a more limited sphere" (1980, 41).

Firms that are stuck in the middle compete at a disadvantage because the cost leaders, differentiators, and focusers are all able to concentrate their capabilities more effectively. Typically, being stuck means that any advantage a firm might have at one point in time is unlikely to be sustained. In addition, firms that are stuck in the middle suffer from a blurred corporate culture, conflicting business activities, and a strained motivation system (1980, 42).

Firms can be stuck in the middle but nevertheless successful. Almost invari-ably, this occurs under circumstances in which other firms in the industry are stuck as well. Ultimately, such firms—and industries—fall into this situation because they failed to make the hard choices about how to compete. Eventually, either firms themselves make those hard choices . . . or the choices are made for them.

Each of the three generic strategies represents a discrete approach to achieving a competitive advantage in the marketplace, and each provides an overall framework for a series of internally consistent actions. No matter how effective the actions, however, a strategy is only successful so long as it enables a firm to resist erosion by the competitive forces that take shape during the course of industry evolution. In some instances, industry evolution will not radically alter the underlying dynamics of the five competitive forces, but in many other instances it will. Understanding this, and knowing whether to stay with or change strategy, is one of the more fundamental issues businesses must face from time to time.

INDUSTRY EVOLUTION, STRUCTURE, AND STRATEGY

Industry evolution is not an inevitable process. The duration of stages varies considerably by industry. In addition, firm behavior affects the tenor of industry evolution. By describing generic industry environments—fragmented, emerging, mature, and declining—Porter's message is not that industry evolution determines strategy, but that structural contexts within industry evolution reflect competitive forces which bear on strategy.

Fragmented Industries[8]

Fragmented industries are those in which no one firm has significant market share. Consequently, there is no single player that can exert strong influence over the industry. Fragmented industries are distinguished by having a large number of small and medium-sized companies. The key point, according to Porter, "is the absence of market leaders with the power to shape industry events" (1980, 191).

---

8 This section draws on Porter, 1980, 191–214.

While fragmentation often exists during "introductory" phases of industry evolution, it is not limited to that period alone. A number of economic factors can cause fragmentation:

- ❑ Low entry barriers.[9]

- ❑ Absence of economies of scale or experience curve.

- ❑ High transportation costs, or constraints, which keep production and distribution local.[10]

- ❑ High inventory costs or erratic sales fluctuations.[11]

- ❑ When size presents no inherent advantage relative to buyers and suppliers.

- ❑ Diseconomies of scale.[12]

- ❑ Exit barriers holding back consolidation.

There is nothing inherent in fragmented industries that requires a particular generic strategy. In formulating any strategy, however, it is important to

---

[9] One reason for fragmentation in the mental health professions is that there are relatively low entry barriers facing psychiatrists, psychologists, psychiatric, and other social workers, as well as various pop therapists. Similar dynamics *had* existed among internists, family physicians, and pediatricians, but increasingly competitive conditions, practice administration costs, and the demands imposed especially by HMO gatekeeper/PCP arrangements have all tended to increase the entry barriers in most typical urban and suburban communities.

[10] This factor contributes to fragmentation in healthcare because patients must go to where the service is produced, and the industry norm is that such locations (e.g., physicians' offices, clinics, and hospitals) be within 20–30 minutes of where people live. In theory, the more patients are able to avail themselves of electronic or "informationalized" linkages to providers, the more concentrated provider organization in healthcare delivery may become, and the more distant patients may be from substantial components of a total delivery system. This point also relates to more widespread reliance on nurse practitioners and physicians assistants. The role that informationalization can play in the doctor-patient relationship is discussed in Chapter 6.

[11] Both of these encourage fragmentation because they undermine the advantages that follow from economies of scale. Large-scale facilities are, in fact, at a disadvantage compared to smaller, nimbler firms. The same can be said for complex, established operations compared to less specialized facilities.

[12] For example, industries where there are rapid product changes, where style changes demand an immediate response, where there are diverse market needs, where low overhead is a critical success variable, or where the product is basically a personal service.

understand 1) the key characteristics of the competitive forces in the fragmented industry, 2) the causes of fragmentation, 3) whether and how fragmentation can be overcome, 4) whether it is profitable to overcome fragmentation, and 5) what the most advantageous position is in a fragmented situation.

Competitive advantage in fragmented industries is most likely achieved by recognizing industry developments early and capitalizing on them before competitors do. Options to *promote consolidation* include 1) making selective acquisitions to achieve a critical mass, 2) separating out those aspects of the industry that reinforce fragmentation from those that do not and concentrating on the latter, and 3) establishing economies of scale plus possibly integrating forward or backward. Options to *cope with fragmentation* include 1) having effective, decentralized management structures, 2) establishing low-cost, standardized capabilities wherever possible, 3) offering value added product or service features, and 4) specializing by product type, market segment, customer, or geographic area.

A major trap in fragmented industries is the lure of undisciplined, opportunistic strategies that expose a firm to increased overhead and competitor retaliation. Successful strategies, on the other hand, build on small, continuous victories, establishing a well-defined competitive advantage over the long term.

Emerging Industries[13]

"Emerging industries are newly formed or reformed industries that have been created by technological innovations, shifts in relative cost relationships, emergence of new consumer needs or other economic and sociological changes." A core characteristic of emerging industries is that there are no "rules of the game." Strategically, the great challenge is to strike the best possible balance between risks inherent in the absence of competitive rules and rewards inherent in what appears to be open-ended opportunities.

Porter describes a series of characteristics commonly associated with emerging industries:

---

[13]This section draws on Porter, 1980, 215–236.

❏ Technological uncertainty.

❏ Strategic uncertainty.

❏ High initial costs but steep cost reductions.

❏ Prominence of newly formed companies.

❏ Prominence of first-time buyers.

❏ Production bottlenecks creating short time horizons.

❏ Corporate and/or government subsidies.

Emerging industries are not distinguished by unusual or especially prohibitive entry barriers. Other factors impacting the competitive forces include 1) inadequate infrastructure (e.g., distribution channels and service capability), 2) lack of product standardization, 3) erratic product quality, 4) customer confusion, 5) relatively high production costs, 6) supplier difficulties, and 7) retaliation from competitor industries.

An overriding goal in the strategic thinking of emerging industries is to exploit the market potential that industry conditions present. One objective should be to promote substitution from older, parallel markets and to achieve market penetration with first-time buyers.[14] A second objective should be to establish industry standards for product quality, marketing, and pricing. Ironically, even though emerging industries represent perhaps the most opportune time for pursuing self-interest, self-interest is best served when competitors also support the industry as a whole.[15] Regardless of whether firms pursue a strategy based on cost leadership, differentiation, or focus, competitive advantage depends on both objectives being achieved.

---

[14]The timing of market penetration is influenced by switching costs, performance and cost advantages, the cost of failure caused by switching, and the threat of obsolescence.

[15]For example, failing to deter substandard quality and fly-by-night producers can set an emerging industry back or even destroy it. In the healthcare industry, this is a major reason for the certification of HMOs and PPOs as well as ambulatory surgery centers (ASCs). Historically, it is also one reason for the various health professions embracing the early 20th century movement toward licensure and certification.

Transition to Maturity[16]

Maturity does not occur at a standard point in an industry's evolution. It can be delayed by innovations or accelerated by external events that are beyond an industry's control. In many firms, management does not recognize the transition to maturity until it is too late. In others, management is aware and plans accordingly.

The transition to industry maturity is signaled by a number of important changes in the competitive forces:

- ❑ Slow growth and increased competition for market share.
- ❑ Greater prominence of experienced, repeat buyers.
- ❑ Competitive issues shifting to cost and service.
- ❑ Topping-out of industry capacity.
- ❑ New product applications becoming harder to come by.
- ❑ Overall industry profit decline.
- ❑ Distributors' margins decreasing while their power increases.

Whereas growth phases tend to mask strategic errors, maturity exposes strategic errors. Some of the greatest difficulties companies confront occur during the transition to maturity. These include 1) older, established self-perceptions obscuring current realities; 2) companies becoming cash traps, with diminished opportunity to recoup investments; 3) companies sacrificing market share too readily for short-term profit; 4) management resenting price competition; 5) management opting for new and better products, rather than selling existing products more competitively; and 6) management refusing to sell off or eliminate excess capacity.

The consequences of being "stuck in the middle" are most apparent during the transition to maturity. Maturity forces companies to clearly choose from among the generic strategies. But regardless of the generic strategy, the most successful approaches involve more functional organization, greater central coordination and control, and reduced overhead. Rigorous cost analysis is important at this juncture, as is adopting process innovations that lower the cost of production. In maturity, companies can gain a competitive advan-

---

[16]This section draws on Porter, 1980, 237–253.

tage by increasing the quantity of goods sold to fewer buyers rather than selling to more buyers. In addition, selling to "good" buyers becomes strategically more important than selling to more buyers.

Declining Industries[17]

The declining phase of industry evolution does not come about because of business cycles or short-term fluctuations in business conditions. Decline is marked by an absolute drop in unit sales over a protracted period and the industry succumbing to product substitution as well as obsolescence. Businesses themselves suffer from falling profits, which in turn cause cutbacks in product lines, R&D, and advertising.

Conditions in declining industries are exacerbated by a variety of developments among the competitive forces. These include 1) a decline in demand caused by technological substitution, shifting customer needs, and/or an absolute reduction in the size of customer groups; 2) elevated exit barriers resulting from high fixed costs, durable or specialized assets, and intractable strategic considerations; and 3) competitive rivalry made worse by parity among existing firms, higher prices from suppliers, and growing dependency on distributors.

Porter describes four options available to firms in declining industries:

- ❑ Leadership.
- ❑ Niche.
- ❑ Harvest.
- ❑ Divestment.

The first option is to *seek leadership*. This option is most likely to be successful with firms that already have a competitive advantage. Tactical steps to establish leadership include:

- ❑ Aggressive pricing and marketing actions to increase share and reduce industry capacity.
- ❑ Selective acquisitions to gain market share and reduce competitor capacity.

17This section draws on Porter, 1980, 254–274.

❏ Demonstrations of superior strength and a strong commitment to the business.

❏ Reducing exit barriers by taking over competitors' contracts and assuming their liabilities.

A second option is to pursue a *niche strategy*. Niche strategies only make sense in declining industries if the target market is stable and long-term demand is projected to show an acceptable rate of return. Also, niche strategies require that a firm establish a defensible position relative to not only more powerful, but potentially more dangerous and unpredictable competitors.

A third option is *harvest*. Not unlike the cash cow described in the Henderson chapter, harvest strategy means milking past strengths. A harvest strategy seeks to earn as much as possible for as long as possible, within the framework of existing operations. Investment and new initiatives are either not pursued at all or kept to a minimum. Tactics might well include reducing the number of products, eliminating smaller customers, using fewer distribution channels, and cutting back on service.

The final option is *divestment*. With divestment, the goal is to exit the industry. Divestment means complete liquidation. The most successful divestments are those that occur sooner rather than later, before the full implications of decline are apparent.

There are at least five variables the strategist should consider in sorting out which option to pursue: 1) whether the industry is heading for a precipitous or gradual decline; 2) what a firm's strengths are compared to the competition; 3) whether there are market segments of value to focus on; 4) whether the industry is changing in ways that pose other opportunities in the future; and 5) whether, given entirely different industries to invest in, staying makes good sense. In declining industries, reading the environment accurately—and early—could well be the difference between survival and failure.

HEALTHCARE INDUSTRY STRUCTURE AND EVOLUTION

Healthcare in the United States is frequently characterized as a "nonsystem." The inference is that the delivery system naturally functions irrationally, unpredictably and in ways that undermine the best efforts of government and the private sector to achieve efficiency and savings. The view that healthcare is a nonsystem is telling because it suggests a penchant for irony over analysis. This section will show how Porter's analysis in *Competitive Strategy* furthers the understanding of healthcare as a *system* and, by extension, poses implications for business strategy in medicine as well as public policy.

Perhaps the best starting point is to turn to one of Porter's five competitive forces: The bargaining power of buyers. Buyers are important because they represent demand. Without demand, there can be no business. When accounting for healthcare's nonsystem qualities, analysts emphasize that demand, particularly as it relates to private health insurance, consists of two kinds of buyers: employer and employee.

Health insurance, be it HMO, PPO, or traditional, is initially sold to the employer. After the employer chooses to offer X, Y, Z plans, employees select one. Given this, the conclusion is drawn that there really is no significant bargaining power on the part of buyers. Employees have insurance that protects them from the full impact of not only provider charges, but the volume of services providers authorize. And employers, notwithstanding concerns about health costs eroding profit margins, often do not want to "rock the boat" with changes that could jeopardize employee relations.[18] For a variety of reasons, then, the bargaining power of buyers is not an especially threatening competitive force in the healthcare system.

The growth of public policy promoting managed competition is directly tied to ineffective demand in healthcare. Since employers and employees do not wield clout as purchasers, the goal of managed competition is to move people into managed care systems and have those systems wield clout as buyers vis-á-vis providers (physicians, hospitals, pharmacies, etc.). With a reinvigorated demand, it is assumed, prices will come down and cost containment will be achieved. The problem with this assumption is that it treats demand too superficially, glossing over the relationship between *industry evolution* and demand on the one hand and *industry structure* and demand on

---

18I have frequently encountered this attitude with senior benefits people from large and medium-sized corporations. In some instances, union considerations preclude change. In others, I have been told that management's "plate is full" with other benefit matters. And on more than one occasion, it was suggested that what looks like a "no brainer" from the outside is "just not that simple" when it comes to implementing health benefit changes for employees.

the other. Within each of these relationships, I would argue, there is an important contradiction. Through Porter's model, both contradictions become apparent.

Contradiction # 1: Cost Containment and Managed Care as an Emerging Industry

This first contradiction is rooted in the relationship between industry evolution and demand. The health insurance industry underwent a series of developments in the 1980s. These developments included: 1) the inability of conventional insurance to curtail healthcare inflation; 2) the continued substitution of ERISA exempt self-insurance for traditional group health insurance; 3) the marketplace pushing commercial carriers (who historically had not been sensitive to controlling healthcare costs) to aggressively pursue cost containment; 4) a revolution in management information systems giving insurance bureaucracies the ability to exercise greater control over providers; and 5) government-led efforts through DRGs and other reimbursement methodologies to change the nature of provider payment.

The cumulative effect of these developments changed the basic character of the health insurance industry. In the 1950–1970 period, for example, health insurance was anything but a growth industry. For commercial carriers it was a loss leader, intended primarily as a way to sell life insurance, pension, and other financial products to corporate America. For the Blues, it was more like a cash cow, positioned primarily around state regulations entitling Blue Cross to a hospital "differential."[19] As a result of the 1980s, though, the health insurance industry changed dramatically.

During the 1980s, *managed care transformed the health insurance industry's life cycle.* Where the industry had been fairly mature up to the beginning of the decade, developments during that decade recast health insurance into an

---

[19]The "differential" is a special hospital discount that states have traditionally given Blue Cross plans in exchange for fulfilling certain community obligations, the two most important being a commitment to insure all individuals regardless of their health condition and to offer a standard community rate for the individual and small group market. The differential once enabled Blue Cross plans to pay hospitals anywhere from 20–40 percent less than commercial carriers. The cost advantage realized from this differential compensated the Blues for the additional costs incurred as a result of their community obligations. During the 1980s, though, most states significantly reduced the differential accorded their Blue Cross plans.

"emerging" industry. The focal point was the growth of managed care and the establishment of new rules, plus product and process innovations that reshaped the nature of health insurance. Despite managed care's commitment to cost containment, therefore, *emerging industry behavior* in health insurance contradicted—and in some ways continues to contradict—managed care's stated goal. Three points stand out here.

First, managed care performance is a function of the industry stage of which it is a part. As mentioned earlier, one facet of emerging industries is that the old rules no longer apply. This bears directly on the approach to profit and loss adopted by health insurers. An actuarial rule of thumb is that the health insurance industry operates in profit and loss cycles of six to seven years. How does that cycle square with managed competition where consumers are expected to "shop" and change plans, when at least one of the core elements of HMOs—health prevention and promotion—requires a long-term time horizon? In addition, how do the assumptions defining profit and loss cycles change given the extensive commingling of capitation and fee-for-service, and the different economies presupposed in each? Part of the answer to both questions is supplied by Porter, who refers to the short-term time horizon of emerging industries, and the pressure to grow at the expense of what is best in the long term for the industry as a whole (1980, 219).

Second, managed care is itself a thriving industry, selling cost containment for profit. Firms comprising this industry produce a wide variety of both high- and low-tech products and services. These firms would be foolish not to be as aggressive as possible for as long as possible while growth opportunities existed. In effect, their success institutionalizes very separate business interests in the markets they serve. The greater their success, the more fiefdoms they create. Rather than managed care bringing about a situation in which the whole is greater than the sum of its parts, each of the parts is much more likely to take on a life of its own. From this perspective, the celebrated nonsystem qualities of the American healthcare system can be attributed to managed care behaving as it should—as an emerging industry.

Third, managed care systems have promoted ambulatory care as a vehicle for cost containment, but that is not how hospitals, physicians, and investors have promoted it. For hospitals, ambulatory care is a way to bill for clinical services on a fee-for-service basis outside of DRGs and per diems. It is also an alternative source of revenue when patients do not require hospitalization. For physicians, ambulatory care is a way to compete against hospitals by capturing portions of the profitable secondary hospital product for themselves. Currently, for instance, almost all testing and surgery in ophthalmology can be performed on an outpatient basis. As the state-of-the-art in procedural technology evolves, other surgical specialties can be expected to follow suit. For outside investors, ambulatory care is where the growth opportunities exist, not only because of increased demand, technology, and the continued prominence of fee-for-service, but also because this sector has been fragmented for so long it is starved for the discipline of corporate organization. In short, rather than controlling costs under managed care, ambulatory care has been a source of increased industry revenues and profit.

Earlier, I discussed Porter's comments about firms being "stuck in the middle." Being stuck means not developing a clear strategy based on either cost, differentiation, or focus. Invariably, firms failing in this regard spread themselves too thin and engage in activities that are at cross-purposes with one another. The performance of such firms is deficient because their costs could be lower, their product features could be stronger, or their appeal to specific customer groups could be more effective. Firms that are stuck operate at a competitive disadvantage. But this is a theoretical disadvantage. Whether others exploit it depends on the effectiveness of their own strategy and on the pressures of the marketplace generated by the stage in the life cycle governing the industry as a whole.

The untold story about the seemingly intractable problems of cost containment in American medicine is that health insurance under managed care is still in an emerging stage of industry evolution, and *the dynamics of this stage not only tolerate but encourage firms being stuck in the middle.* Porter describes this situation as one of "strategic uncertainty" where "No 'right' strategy has been clearly identified, and different firms are groping with different approaches to product/market positioning, marketing, servicing and so on."[20] The implication for healthcare policy is that cost containment will not be achieved until managed care health insurance progresses to a point in indus-

---

[20]Porter, 1980, 217. That industry behavior is both groping and tolerant of firms being stuck in the middle is evident with just a casual glance at the managed care map, which includes staff, group, direct contract, indirect contract, IPA, and PHO model HMOs; gatekeeper, out-of-panel, and point-of-service arrangements; and EPOs as well as PPOs with and without gatekeepers.

try evolution where firms can no longer be stuck in the middle and still grow. The implication for business strategy is that this point be reached before government tries to impose it.

Contradiction # 2: Managed Competition and the Medical Profession

This second contradiction is rooted in the relationship between industry structure and demand. As mentioned in Chapter 4, managed competition is a policy that relies on a *demand strategy* to stimulate the growth of market forces in healthcare delivery. At the heart of this policy is the institutionalization of what in Porter's language is the bargaining power of buyers in the marketplace. Through the use of purchasing cooperatives, business group coalitions, or other formally organized alliances, the assumption is that individuals and small businesses will be able to obtain competitive premiums from managed care health plans with the same ease and buying power as larger employers, and that competition for enrollees among plans will encourage more cost-effective medicine.[21]

There is an interesting analogy between the role of purchasing cooperatives, coalitions, and alliances under managed competition and the role of health

---

[21]As of this writing, purchasing alliances organized specifically to negotiate discounts from insurers either exist or are being developed in at least 25 states. For discussions on various purchasing initiatives see, for example, John Fialka. "Washington State Healthcare Package Sets Up an Early Test for Clinton Ideas." *The Wall Street Journal* (April 12, 1993): B3; George Anders. "States Slow Ambitious Healthcare Reform Moves But Continue to Act as Laboratories of Innovation." *The Wall Street Journal* (July 8, 1994): A12; Larry Rohter. "Employers in Orlando Create an Envied Model." *New York Times* (June 30, 1994); Ron Winslow. "Market Forces Are Starting to Produce Significant Cuts in Healthcare Costs." *The Wall Street Journal* (June 21, 1994): A2; Lisa Scott. "St. Louis Businesses Form Buying Group." *Modern Healthcare* (August 22, 1994): 7; and Christine Woolsey. "Illinois Employers to Form Health Alliance." *Business Insurance* (September 19, 1994): 77. Two excellent descriptions of managed competition are The White House Domestic Policy Council. *The President's Health Security Plan* (Times Books, 1993); and Alain C. Enthoven. *Managed Competition in Healthcare Financing and Delivery*, prepared under a grant by the Robert Wood Johnson Foundation, January 13, 1993, and considered "mandatory reading" for the Clinton Administration healthcare task force. Also see A. Enthoven. "The History and Principles of Managed Competition." *Health Affairs* 12 (1993): 24–48; and A. Enthoven and R. Kronic. "A Consumer Choice Health Plan for the 1990s: Universal Health Insurance in a System Designed to Promote Quality and Economy." *New England Journal of Medicine* 320 (January 5 and 12, 1989): 29–37 and 94–101.

systems agencies (HSAs) in the health planning legislation of the 1970s. While HSAs are now all but defunct, their role was to discipline the *supply* side of healthcare delivery by making recommendations to state health planning agencies for or against certificates of need (CONs). These CONs were needed before capital expenditures over a certain dollar amount would be approved. The assumption behind CONs was that by limiting the supply of major capital expenditures in a market, there would be an absolute limit on the utilization of expensive or unnecessary services and that such limits would help contain the excesses of fee-for-service medicine.

With managed competition, the role of purchasing cooperatives is to discipline the *demand* side of healthcare delivery so market forces stimulate the growth of managed care systems. The interest in promoting managed care systems is that they link healthcare financing with delivery. By increasing their market share, it is assumed, providers, particularly physicians, will be forced to join HMOs, PPOs, and other health plans that deliver medical services more economically.

The difficulties I anticipate with this demand strategy parallel the difficulties experienced under the older regulatory strategies of the 1970s. In the same way that regulations bearing on supply could not substitute for competitive initiatives, which critics argued had to come from the marketplace, regulations bearing on demand, I would argue, cannot substitute for *integration initiatives*, which also have to come from the marketplace. For managed care systems to succeed, it will have to be through the integration of healthcare financing and delivery in the marketplace, not through a reorganization of the demand function created as an artifact of health policy. Health policy may facilitate the growth of managed care systems, but it is *business strategy in those systems* that will determine whether and to what degree managed competition is effective.

What advocates of managed competition forget, and what those who determine managed care business strategy must remember, is that they are *trying to industrialize an industry that was never industrialized.* The central issue in all of this is the role of physicians. Perhaps the greatest political achievement of the American medical profession this century is that it circumscribed physician autonomy and authority in such a way that physicians have never been threatened by the backward integration of health insurers. The separate institutional spheres of physicians and insurers, buyers and suppliers respectively, has always been maintained.[22] In my judgment, managed competition will not succeed until the relationship between those spheres is rethought and *new forms of integration in the production of health services* are adopted. Combining financing and delivery systems to accommodate a reinvigorated demand for health services will not suffice. Indeed, absent efforts to achieve new forms of integration in production, problems associated with inflation, quality, and access will not only worsen under managed competition, they may well become more difficult to solve.

Those who think managed competition will gradually solve the healthcare system's inflationary spiral, neglect three problems that persist even under current managed care systems:

❑ First, as is widely recognized, discount fee-for-service in both HMOs and PPOs increases rather than decreases the perverse incentive that has plagued traditional health insurance. This is reflected in various "gaming" strategies physicians resort to in order to compensate for lost income: 1) churning, which refers to performing more procedures, ordering more tests, and scheduling more frequent revisits than is really necessary; 2) gouging, which refers to the decision to perform certain diagnostic tests and procedures solely on the basis of whether or not they are reimbursed by insurance; and 3) CPT creep, which involves inflating what was done in the physician's office to maximize reimbursement in the billing process.[23]

❑ Second, capitating physicians in HMOs has its own perverse incentive: Doing less rather than more. This includes 1) avoiding tests which economically may not be cost-effective, but clinically might identify an unlikely problem; 2) putting off patients' needed and inevitable surgery

---

[22]Notable exceptions to this pattern include Kaiser Permanente in California, Group Health of Puget Sound in Seattle, Harvard Community Health Plan in Boston, Geisinger Health Plan in Pennsylvania, and the Health Insurance Plan (HIP) in New York.

[23]*Consumer Reports* (July 1992) estimated that $130 billion was the annual national cost of unnecessary procedures and services. While not all of the $130 billion can be attributed to churning, gouging, and CPT creep, if you assume one half, then at least 8 percent of the approximately $800 billion spent for healthcare in 1992 can be attributed to these factors. I have been told by one very well-informed physician overseeing physician utilization in one specialty network that at least 40 percent in his specialty are involved in some form of gaming the system.

for as long as possible; 3) restricting patient referrals to specialists or, what I have frequently seen, sending referrals to the "generalists" of a specialty rather than the appropriate subspecialist; and 4) having PCP/gatekeepers make the final decision about treatment by specialists and subspecialists.[24]

❑ Third, with the exception of simply rationing, systems of managed care have demonstrated no special capacity for controlling the inflationary pressures of high-tech medicine.[25] This is not to say that managed care systems have not slowed down the rate of inflation. It is to say, however, that they have implemented no new or unique principles of organization. I believe it is here that the consequences of not rethinking the relationships between the institutional spheres of suppliers and buyers, physicians, and insurers—not rethinking relationships of integration *at the level of production*—spell the most trouble for the long-term prospects of managed care systems and the efficacy of managed competition as health policy.

What is absolutely essential to accept about the enterprise of "medicine" is that it is an *acute, episodic enterprise by nature* and that from a strictly cost/benefit standpoint, medicine is inherently not cost-effective. If we think in terms of a numerator and denominator, with the numerator being a sick individual and the denominator being a total population, medicine is ultimately about treating the numerator. It will always be a more cost-effective use of health resources to invest in the denominator as opposed to the numerator, in programs geared to the health of total populations rather than

---

[24]For an excellent commentary on this last point from a consumer's point of view, see Susan Rosenfeld. "So You Want to Join an HMO? Good Luck." *New York Times* (August 9, 1994): A23.

[25]A recent case study is a situation reported in Miami, one of the more concentrated managed care markets nationally. Two hospitals located within minutes of each other each have a gamma knife at a cost of $3 million. The second hospital purchased the knife despite the fact that this device can treat only a few types of tumors and demand in that market does not justify the supply. As reported in *The Wall Street Journal*, "By some estimates, just six of them could have treated all American patients last year." Instead, physicians in the two Miami hospitals, as well as physicians across the country, are clamoring for this "new medical status symbol"—and hospitals, notwithstanding pressures from HMOs and PPOs, are expected to oblige them. See George Anders. "Hospital Rush to Buy A $3 Million Device Few Patients Can Use." *The Wall Street Journal* (April 20, 1994): A1.

the individual. Of course, from witch doctor to modern physician, society has always sanctioned the legitimacy of this not-so-cost-effective enterprise. The significance of high-tech medicine, however, is that it exacerbates the problem of cost/benefit exponentially. The more high-tech medicine becomes, the less cost-effective it is because the resource expenditures are at the margin where the costs are higher and the success often less predictable and less long term.

I am not suggesting that any of this is bad. Indeed, I believe progress in high-tech medicine is an indice of our progress as a civilization. It should be something Americans are proud of. But high-tech medicine also has to be organized, and it is here that the real conflict between the medical profession and managed competition exists.

There is a tendency to view this conflict as one between the profession's long-standing independence on the one hand, and managed care bureaucracies with their penchant for control on the other. Where once the medical profession stood for physician independence and autonomy, physicians are now overwhelmed by the second-guessing of their clinical decisions and a heap of paperwork they are required to perform. I would argue, however, it is not the frustration physicians feel that goes to the core of the conflict between the medical profession and managed competition, but the inconsistency between the model of production the profession continues to be predicated on and the model of production managed care systems have so far established.

Physician frustration is as much a symptom of managed care systems not having effectively integrated the physician role in the production of health services, as is the persistence of healthcare inflation. Indeed, physician frustration and healthcare inflation may be two sides of the same proverbial coin. The fact that rationing in some form is widely accepted as the *modus operandi* for ultimately controlling healthcare inflation is a measure of how inadequately integrated the physician role really is under most of managed care.

For this reason, I do not believe the policy of managed competition will ever truly succeed until strategic thinking in managed care identifies new functions, new technical responsibilities, and new economic spaces for physicians in the production of health services. What is needed, in other words, is not just the "integration of financing and delivery," which supporters of managed competition advocate, but a transformation in the relationships between suppliers and buyers in the healthcare's industry structure, and one that is particularly suited for the *production requirements of healthcare services in an age of high-tech medicine.* Porter's discussion of the "value chain" in his second major work, *Competitive Advantage,* provides a useful starting point for such strategic thinking.

THE VALUE CHAIN

Satisfying buyer needs is a prerequisite for being successful in business but in itself is not sufficient. Capturing the value created for buyers also should occur. As Porter points out, "Value is what buyers are willing to pay for, and superior value stems from offering lower prices than competitors for equivalent benefits or providing unique benefits that more than offset a higher price" (1985, 3). "Value activities" are the building blocks by which a firm creates a product or service for buyers. The "value chain" is a basic concept in the management literature, and it is used by Porter as a tool for diagnosing problems in the creation of value and finding ways to create and sustain the production of value.

The value chain consists of a series of nine generic value activities. Porter divides these activities into two different categories: Primary activities and support.[26] Primary activities are directly involved in the production of value. They include:

- ❑ **Inbound Logistics.** "Activities associated with receiving, storing and disseminating inputs to the product."

- ❑ **Operations.** "Activities associated with transforming inputs into the final product form."

- ❑ **Outbound Logistics.** "Activities associated with collecting, storing and physically distributing the product to buyers."

- ❑ **Marketing and Sales.** "Activities associated with providing a means by which buyers can purchase the product and inducing them to do so."

- ❑ **Service.** "Activities associated with providing service to enhance or maintain the value of the product."

---

[26]The definitions below are taken from Porter, 1985, 39–43.

Support activities are indirectly involved in the production of value. Their contributions extend in different ways to the value chain as a whole. Support activities include:

❑ **Procurement.** Activities associated with the function of purchasing inputs.

❑ **Technology Development.** Activities associated with the development of techniques, know-how, and technical procedures.

❑ **Human Resource Management.** Activities associated with recruiting, hiring, training, developing, and compensating personnel.

❑ **Firm Infrastructure.** Activities associated with management, planning, finance, accounting, legal, government affairs, and quality control.

The value chain and generic value activities are described in Figure 5–2.

Figure 5–2.   The Generic Value Chain

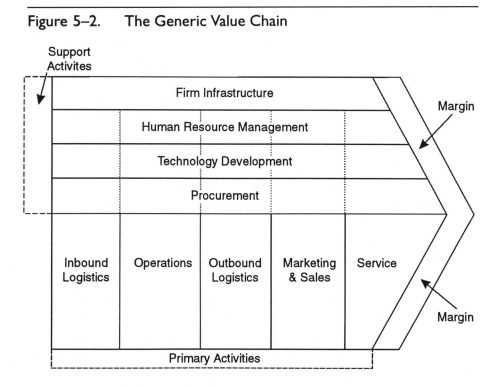

Source: Reprinted with the permission of The Free Press, a Division of Simon & Schuster from *Competitive Advantage: Creating and Sustaining Superior Performance* by Michael E. Porter. Copyright © 1985 by Michael E. Porter.

While the value chain refers to a firm, Porter emphasizes that it is also "embedded in a larger stream of activities," what he calls the "value system" of an industry. That is, in all industries, suppliers have value chains, as do channels and buyers, and all of these value chains are related to each other.

According to Porter, "Gaining and sustaining a competitive advantage depends on understanding not only a firm's value chain but how the firm fits in the overall value system" (1985, 34). Strategic thinking should reflect how a firm's value chain compares to competitors and how the firm's value chain compares to the value system in its industry. Value activities should be analyzed with a view to both the firm's performance as well as the trends, issues, and strategies operating within the larger industry value system. Differences among competitor value chains, and differences in how competitors' value chains perform vis-á-vis an industry's value system, can be a major source of competitive advantage (1985, 36, 45).

To build a competitive advantage, it is necessary for firms to define their value chain. Defining the value chain involves isolating activities with discrete functions. According to Porter, "The basic principle is that activities should be isolated and separated that 1) have different economics, 2) have a high potential impact on differentiation, or 3) represent a significant or growing proportion of cost" (1985, 45). In addition, Porter suggests that firms need to identify key value activities for strategic investment and possibly redefine routine activities as key.

While superior value activities enable one firm to achieve a competitive advantage over another, Porter emphasizes not so much the independence, but the interdependence of these activities. Often, it is the interdependence or linkages between value activities, rather than an individual value activity, that gives a firm its competitive advantage. Linkages create an opportunity for firms to increase efficiency and reduce costs. They can exist between value activities within a firm or between a firm's value chain and the value chains of suppliers and channels. These are vertical linkages. Vertical linkages with suppliers raises the possibility of reducing the zero sum quality between supplier and buyer. Vertical linkages with channels create additional value that is not only shared by the firm and channel, but is ultimately passed on directly or indirectly to the buyer (1985, 48–52).

THE VALUE CHAIN AND COMPETITIVE ADVANTAGE

The value chain is the framework of a firm Porter suggests management should use to build either of the two types of competitive advantage: Cost leadership or differentiation. The application of the value chain to each is described below.

Cost Leadership

A firm achieves cost leadership if it produces the same product as its competitors at a lower cost or produces a better product than its competitors at the same cost. "A firm's cost position results from the cost behavior of its value activities" (1985, 70). Cost behavior is determined by what Porter calls "cost drivers." Whether or not a firm is able to establish cost leadership depends on the impact of cost drivers in its value chain compared to cost drivers in value chains of competitors. The significance of any one cost driver will vary by firm as well as by industry circumstances. Porter describes 10 major cost drivers:[27]

- ❏ **Economies of Scale.** Economies of scale result from the ability to perform activities more efficiently at a larger volume or to amortize the variable cost of such activities as advertising and R&D over a greater sales volume. Economies of scale are realized not only through technological capacity employed in value activities, but in how a firm organizes its value activities.

- ❏ **Learning.** Learning includes such factors as improved efficiencies, enhanced design modifications, simplified scheduling, a smarter use of personnel, and streamlined work flows. If learning is proprietary, the cost advantage that results is likely to be sustainable. When there is spillover to the industry, what was a cost advantage for a firm can end up lowering costs for the industry overall.

- ❏ **Pattern of Capacity Utilization.** When a firm has substantial fixed costs, successful performance is significantly affected by capacity utili-

---

[27]The definitions below draw on Porter, 1985, 70–83.

zation. The higher the fixed costs, the higher the penalty for underutilization. Firms with high fixed costs and stable utilization derive significant cost advantages if competitors with high fixed costs have inconsistent utilization.

❑ **Linkages.** As discussed above, linkages provide an opportunity to lower costs and improve the coordination between related functions. Linkages can be between two value activities within a firm or between value chains of a firm and suppliers and/or channels (vertical linkages). Firms with significant vertical linkages have the potential to realize a major cost advantage.

❑ **Interrelationships.** Interrelationships result from one unit of a firm sharing a value activity or know-how with another unit. When one of two competing firms is part of a diversified business and is able to exploit a sister unit's capabilities, that firm has the potential to realize an important cost advantage. One danger, though, is that the borrowed capacity may not be the best, or it may have hidden weaknesses that only become apparent after it is too late.

❑ **Integration.** Integration refers to a firm either developing in-house capacity to produce certain inputs or acquiring such capacity. Integration can lower costs by eliminating the need to contend with market prices and the bargaining power of suppliers. Potential risks of integration involve inflexibility within a firm's value chain and not performing a function as well or as economically compared to outside suppliers.

❑ **Timing.** Being first in a market lowers the cost of establishing a brand identity. In addition, it can lower the scale required and, therefore, operational costs. Late movers also derive significant cost advantages, however. They can benefit from competitor mistakes, lower product development costs, and being in a position to target specific market segments.

❑ **Discretionary Policies Independent of Other Cost Drivers.** Costs of value activities can be affected by decisions having nothing to do with other cost drivers. Examples include decisions on the kinds of buyers served (large or small), channels to work through (few or many), and adopting process and technology innovations. Firms making discretionary policies with an eye to how they affect cost behavior in the value chain achieve a cost advantage over competitors prone to bold decisions without regard to cost.

❑ **Location.** Cost factors stemming from location include wages, cost of living, access to skilled and unskilled personnel, transportation, marketing, local culture, and logistical factors. Often, wages and taxes are the immediate considerations when evaluating the cost of a location. Technological developments and innovative vertical linkages, however, could have a far more significant impact on cost.

❑ **Institutional Factors.** Institutional factors are frequently beyond the control of an individual firm. They include taxes, laws, regulations, utility costs, and political pressures. Insofar as one firm is able to influence institutional factors, competing firms are likely to be at a disadvantage.

In addition to "cost drivers" within a firm, Porter refers to the "cost dynamics" of an industry. These include 1) changes in industry growth, 2) changes in industry cost behavior, 3) different industry learning rates, 4) different technological changes, 5) inflation, 6) aging, and 7) market adjustments. Firms that identify changes in the cost dynamics of their industry and adjust their value chain before their competitors, are in a position to build a cost advantage.

Building a cost advantage requires that selected cost drivers be in place to lower costs in the value chain. Porter suggests that the most important drivers for a cost advantage are 1) economies of scale, 2) interrelationships, 3) linkages, 4) proprietary learning, and 5) policy choices to create proprietary product or process technology. Building a sustainable cost advantage requires not only that cost drivers be in place, though. Sustainability depends on the impact of cost drivers on value activities and their relationships within the overall value chain. "Cost leaders usually accumulate cost advantages gained from numerous sources in the value chain that interact and reinforce each other." For Porter, as for Henderson, then, it is this cumulative and interactive quality that makes a cost leader's approach difficult for competitors to duplicate (1985, 112–113).

Differentiation

"Differentiation" is not the same as "different." Firms can be different, but not differentiated. Differentiation depends on a firm's capacity to be unique at something of value to buyers beyond simply low price. Value is central to any differentiation strategy. Porter emphasizes that value does not stem just from physical product or marketing. It can be produced anywhere in a firm's value chain (1985, 119).

On a related point, he also emphasizes that the costs associated with differentiation play a critical role in the buyer's value equation. Since a buyer has to weigh the benefits of what a seller offers against the costs, if the price premium of a product exceeds the benefit, the buyer may not purchase the product. Firms pursuing a differentiation strategy that fail to exploit opportunities to lower costs will lose their advantage when lower-priced competitors match their offering. Conversely, firms that are able to lower their costs can potentially increase demand and create entry barriers deterring competitors. For this reason, cost drivers can be very important to the overall success of a firm's differentiation strategy. According to Porter, the most important cost drivers for differentiation are 1) the key policy choices a firm makes on such matters as product, marketing, technology, and service; 2) linkages established inside and/or outside the firm; and 3) timing (1985, 128–129).

Differentiation ultimately depends on how a firm connects with the buyer's value chain. A successfully differentiated product or service has to create value for the buyer within the framework of the buyer's value chain. "[T]he value a firm creates for its buyer is determined by the whole array of links between the firm's value chain and its buyer's value chain" (1985, 133).

Differentiation creates value for buyers in one of two basic ways: By lowering a buyer's cost, or by raising a buyer's performance. It is the buyer's *perception* of what the seller offers on either of these two counts that is the all-important factor a firm has to address. Porter uses the term "signals of value" to refer to the frame of reference buyer's use in determining perceived value. In many instances, the signals of value a firm appeals to are as important, if not more important, than the actual value a firm creates. "A firm that delivers only modest value but signals it more effectively may actually command a higher price than a firm that delivers higher value but signals it poorly" (1985, 39). Understanding the value a firm creates for a buyer, as well as the signals of value a buyer uses to judge value, are both central to effective differentiation.

Signals of value can be considered the emotional buttons a firm pushes in the buyer. To push them effectively, Porter suggests, firms have to meet two different buyer purchasing criteria: (1985, 142)

- **Use Criteria.** "Purchase criteria that stem from the way in which a supplier affects actual buyer value through lowering buyer cost or raising buyer performance."
- **Signaling Criteria.** "Purchase criteria that stem from signals of value, or means used by the buyer to infer or judge what a supplier's actual value is."

Where use criteria refer to objective considerations of buyer value in the buyer's value chain, signaling criteria refer to subjective considerations and themes associated with such factors as prestige, packaging, reputation, and appearance. Use criteria are important if a firm wants to emphasize its product or the system by which it delivers and supports its product. Signaling criteria are important when buyers have a difficult time measuring a supplier's performance. Signaling criteria can be especially important for firms providing professional services. The more successful any firm is in meeting both criteria, the more successful its appeal to buyers. "Addressing use criteria without also addressing signaling criteria . . . will undermine a buyer's perception of a firm's value. Addressing signaling criteria without meeting use criteria will . . . usually not succeed because buyers will eventually realize that their substantive needs have gone unmet" (1985, 143–145).

Porter describes four approaches that singly or in combination have been used by successful differentiators:[28]

- **Enhance the sources of uniqueness:** 1) develop as many sources of differentiation within the value chain as possible; 2) ensure through design modification, training, and upgrades that the actual product is consistent with the buyer's intended use; 3) employ signals of value to reinforce differentiation; and 4) bundle information with the product, such as special software or continuous readouts, to facilitate buyer value awareness.

---

[28]The four approaches summarized below draw on Porter, 1985, 154–158.

❑ **Make the cost of differentiation an advantage:** 1) exploit all sources of differentiation that are not costly; 2) minimize the cost of differentiation by developing efficiencies, focusing on cost drivers, and reducing signaling costs; 3) leverage all value activities where the firm has a cost advantage; and 4) cut back on costs that have little or no bearing on buyer value.

❑ **Change the rules to create uniqueness:** 1) work through decision makers who are in the best position to appreciate the firm's value; 2) identify and promote unrecognized purchase criteria; and 3) anticipate new developments involving buyers and/or the marketplace.

❑ **Reconfigure the value chain to be unique in entirely new ways:** 1) identify new distribution channels or selling approaches; 2) integrate forward and/or backward to rework channel and/or supplier relationships; and 3) adopt innovative approaches to operations and process technology.

For Porter, formulating strategy based on differentiation involves: 1) understanding who the real buyer is; 2) analyzing the firm's impact on the buyer's value chain; 3) addressing the buyer's purchasing criteria; 4) identifying and evaluating the cost of existing and potential sources of differentiation; 5) determining areas where reducing costs will have a minimal impact on differentiation; 6) establishing the best possible combination of value activities that achieve both differentiation and savings; and 7) pursuing options that are sustainable (1985, 162–163).

PRODUCTION AND CONTROL IN MANAGED CARE

Earlier this century, one of the founding fathers of sociology, Emile Durkheim, drew a classic distinction between two different forms of "social solidarity."[29] The first, attributed to primitive society, was "mechanical." The second, attributed to modern society, was "organic." Durkheim's distinction is useful because it highlights why Porter's work on the value chain is relevant to current developments in managed care.

---

[29]Emile Durkheim. *The Division of Labor* (New York: The Free Press, 1964).

Briefly, mechanical solidarity is *forced solidarity*. In primitive society, social organization turned on a not-so-subtle combination of rigid hierarchy and ritual. Ritual prevented deviation, and rigid hierarchy maintained order. As a result, the economy of primitive society was not prone to innovation and change. Organic solidarity, on the other hand, is *functional solidarity*. While ritual exists in modern society, social organization turns on functional integration in the evolution of a division of labor. Because of the shift from force to function in organizing principles, Durkheim suggested, the economies of modern society are naturally much more open to innovation and change.

These two types of solidarity are what social scientists call "ideal types." For heuristic purposes, they are mentioned because they underscore how principles of organization can be congruent, or incongruent, with the thing being organized. Turning to managed care and managed competition, I would argue that perhaps *the* key issue confronting policy makers, physicians, and patients alike, is whether the principles of organization in various managed systems are themselves congruent or incongruent with the practice and profession of medicine.

From different perspectives, both Porter and Durkheim make the point that with increased complexity, organizational structures need to evolve to satisfy changing functional demands. For Porter, this is reflected in firms changing their value activities as well as the basic configuration of their value chain. For Durkheim, it is reflected negatively—in systems overcompensating and imposing burdensome controls when required changes do not occur. In the first case, principles of organization evolve to meet the functional requirements imposed by a more complex environment; in the latter case, they do not. It is this latter case, I believe, that characterizes much of what is now occuring in American medicine under managed care today.

There are three issues to keep in mind here. The first is that managed care is not new: PPOs can be traced back to the 1930s and the original Blue Cross model of service contracts with "par" or "participating" hospitals; HMOs were first started during World War II when Kaiser Steel provided comprehensive coverage to its employees under a fixed budget; and utilization review evolved during the 1970s when Congress mandated PSROs (Professional Service Review Organizations) to combat overutilization in Medicare. Managed care in its various forms, then, has been a part of the existing healthcare system for half a century. While it has certainly caused changes to healthcare delivery, those changes have been absorbed within the system, preserving, in effect, the underlying logic of fee-for-service medicine.

Second, advocates of managed competition make an enormous leap of faith when they claim that systems of managed care create efficiencies that fee-for-service prevented. The leap follows from the assumption that integrating financing and delivery gives managed care systems the "capability to plan and manage processes of care across the total spectrum of inpatient, outpatient, office and home.[30] This capability does not necessarily translate into more efficient medical practice, however. The problem is that most systems of managed care continue to embrace the model of production inherent in traditional health insurance. With the exception of staff and salaried group model HMOs, managed care systems are still organized to provide healthcare on a *piece-rate basis*. The model of production operating under managed care is not unlike the model of production the medical profession has always employed—that of independent artisans and craftsmen. Physician income is tied to units of service performed, and physician productivity is defined by the number of patients seen in a given time period.

Third, *the piece-rate logic underlying most managed care systems puts medicine and managed care on an inevitable collision course.* Since gains in productivity mean greater volume, the more "productive" physicians are, the more managed care systems will have to pay—and the more they pay, the more control they will be forced to exert. These relationships are compounded by an aging population and the continued growth of costly, high-tech medicine. From this standpoint, the purpose of utilization management is to serve as a control system to curb physician behavior. Notwithstanding physician excesses in testing and procedures, under piece-rate production this control system can be expected to become increasingly adversarial over time.

Going back to Durkheim, then, what I am suggesting is that *managed care's organizational capabilities in the production of health services have not kept pace with the clinical capabilities of medicine. The incongruence between managed care's "cost containment" imperative and piece-rate production has turned much*

30Alain C. Enthoven. *Managed Competition in Healthcare Financing and Delivery*, prepared under a grant by The Robert Wood Johnson Foundation, unpublished, used by the Clinton healthcare task force. (January 13, 1993): 21.

of managed care into essentially bureaucratic control systems designed to reduce volume. These control systems compensate for more advanced forms of physician integration that have yet to evolve. They represent a "mechanical" integration of physicians, where "organic" integration should exist instead. Porter's value chain, I believe, is central to understanding many of the key issues associated with achieving a more functionally driven integration.

Before turning to Porter, though, there are two general points I want to make. First, I am not suggesting that increased piece-rate productivity is bad. I'm suggesting that volume should not be the only measure of productivity. *Value* should also be considered. Where volume is tied to a piece-rate logic, value is tied to what might be called "actuarial logic"—a logic that links the impact of health services on a discrete population to a fixed budget. In *shifting from a volume to a value standard,* piece-rate productivity can then be subsumed within a broader production function. The challenge presupposed in this broader production function is to have the full armamentarium of medical services structured and organized so that a given population receives the absolute highest quality healthcare possible under budget. In colloquial terms, it is a challenge for medical resources to be working not just "harder" but "smarter."

Second, a deep-seated microeconomic bias shapes most of the prevailing thinking on managed competition. That bias turns on the determinate role ascribed to incentives over structure in changing how healthcare services are delivered. While supporters of HMOs, for example, assume that financial incentives under capitation will motivate changes in production, I would argue that changes in structure have to occur at the level of production first. Relying on capitation to stimulate changes in production is like leaving children alone in the forest to develop their survival skills. Perhaps the greatest strategic challenge senior executives in the managed care industry face today is to change the structure of production in healthcare delivery before changes in financial incentives, such as global budgets, capitation, case rates and other prepaid arrangements, fully take hold.

THE VALUE CHAIN AND MANAGED CARE

Unlike other industries, the concept of "production" has never had a particularly strong resonance in the health services industry. In part, this is because of the episodic quality of healthcare. In part, it is because of the authority wielded by the medical profession. And in part, it is because of the plethora of stakeholders that dominate American medicine. Consequently, rather than "production," the term "delivery system" is typically used. Hence, the current call for a "more efficient delivery system." But an efficient delivery system addresses interaction among parts, not what is produced by the whole. The widespread belief in government and the private sector that managed care will bring about a more efficient delivery system reminds me of the comment made by Tregoe and Zimmerman that if an organization is headed in the wrong direction, it doesn't pay to get there any quicker. For this reason, I would add two of Porter's core concepts to the standard lexicon in managed care: "Production of value" and "value chain."

When Porter refers to value, he does so from the standpoint of competitive advantage. Competitive advantage grows out of the value firms create for buyers that exceed the cost of production. Superior value is reflected in firms producing either equivalent benefits at lower prices or unique benefits that justify higher prices. How firms produce either of these two types of value—that is, whether they are producing from the standpoint of cost leadership or differentiation—is dependent on their value chain and the relationship of their value chain to the broader value system. These constructs apply directly to managed healthcare.

Production of Value

In the last section, I drew a distinction between production driven by a volume standard and production driven by a value standard. I suggested that the former is governed by a piece-rate logic; the latter, governed by an actuarial logic. Where volume has been the predominate production standard in healthcare up to now, value, I believe, should become the predominant standard. With value as the standard, the perspective on production changes from the number of patients seen or cases treated to patients seen or cases treated at what level of quality, with what resources, and with what results.

If managed care systems are to be oriented to the production of value, cost of production is certainly important. But *approach* to production is no less important. While payors and providers find it exceedingly difficult to understand their "true" costs, they are still in a position to rethink their approach to production. That is, they can still ask: All right, if I'm producing my services this way and my total cost is approximately X, how can I produce either 1) the same product at a lower cost, or 2) a better product at the same approximate cost?

It is around this point that I believe the managed care industry is at a crossroad. On the one hand, past systems of open-ended reimbursement did not encourage patients, providers, or for that matter even payors to be oriented to a value standard. On the other hand, the limits inherent in current systems of fixed reimbursement—capitation, case rates, and discount fee schedules—require it. As managed care comes under the orbit of fixed reimbursement, more will be expected for less: More services will be demanded by an aging population; more technology will be expected; and more in the way of acute episodic care will be required. Under these circumstances, value becomes *the* critical success factor. Indeed, it may well be that until strategic thinking under managed care focuses squarely on the production of value, quality of healthcare in the United States will deteriorate.

Unfortunately, there is a tendency in managed care to neglect the production of value. One reason is that physicians historically have been reimbursed based on charges. As a result, cost-containment pressures have pushed payors to *extract* discounts from providers. The greater the cost containment pressure, the greater the discounts extracted. Some time ago, for example, I facilitated a meeting between a radiology practice and an HMO to discuss a proposal for an exclusive capitation arrangement. Since the practice had been burned by excessive MRI and CT volume under a capitation contract from another HMO, the meeting was intended to formulate an arrangement that would avoid past mistakes. This particular HMO's reaction, though, was to be as economically "tough" as the competitor and to "get not one penny less of a discount." There really was no interest in developing *a more productive approach*. Later that day, the client I met with, and another, talked to me about selling their practice and getting out of medicine entirely. These, I hasten to add, were top-of-the-line practices with superb credentials and impeccable reputations.

A second reason producing value is neglected under managed care is that the much-vaunted "integration" managed care systems were supposed to achieve has not amounted to very much in the way of *new* integration at all. Hospitals may purchase medical practices, medical practices may consolidate, and traditional insurers may merge with HMOs or PPOs, but these developments have not led to forms of integration that change the approach to production. We are not seeing, to use Porter's word, a "reconfiguration" in how the production process in medical care is organized. As a result, a kind of thermidorian reaction has accompanied the managed care revolution in healthcare, with the *extraction of discounts holding sway over the production of value.*

Value Chain

Managed care preceded managed competition in health policy and, barring a single-payor system, it will continue to evolve no matter what health policy is in the future. Managed care reflects developments in industry evolution involving payors and providers that are intended to achieve cost containment. Anyone who works with physicians, however, understands the depth of their frustration with these developments. I say this not to defend physicians, but to emphasize that until they are effectively integrated *as a part of natural industry evolution under managed care*, expectations regarding cost containment will not be fulfilled. In my judgment, health policy cannot make this integration come about; only business strategy can.

The strains physicians (and hospitals) experience with managed care result from business strategy not having achieved the kinds of integration required for the production of greater value. In fact, the legitimacy that rationing has in the discourse of managed care underscores how far removed the healthcare industry is from realizing genuine breakthroughs in production. Until those breakthroughs are achieved, a financial noose will continue to dominate medicine under managed care. Porter's discussion on the value chain puts all of this in relief.

The trend towards consolidation that started with hospitals in the 1980s has extended to physicians in the 1990s. Among hospitals, consolidation revolved around the formation of multihospital systems. These systems centralized such corporate functions as information management, purchasing, finance, and marketing, all with the goal of achieving greater economies of scale. Physicians are currently undergoing a similar transformation. While the form of this consolidation varies by market, the goal is the same: To achieve greater economies of scale. Porter makes the point, though, and I believe it is especially significant here, that economies of scale have to do with *changes in the way activities are performed* and that economies of scale are to be distinguished from spreading fixed costs over greater volume. "Economies of scale arise from the ability to perform activities differently and more efficiently at a larger volume. . . ." (1985, 71). Spreading fixed costs results in savings, but not necessarily efficiencies in actual performance. Mistaking the former for the latter leads to false conclusions about the functional gains actually realized with the consolidation among hospitals and physicians.

Pushing this theme further, Porter also emphasizes that not all economies of scale are equivalent, and that *strategy should focus on those value activities whose sensitivity to scale will have the greatest impact on performance.* In that context, what is interesting about current concerns for cost containment in healthcare is the focus on administration and claims processing. While there is certainly no disputing that inefficiency exists here, by far the greatest inflationary pressures involve medical practice itself. From Porter's perspective, competitive advantage should be realized by those managed care systems that leverage economies of scale and other cost drivers *within medical practice.*

Figure 5–3 depicts the continuum of managed care systems operating in the healthcare industry today. As the arrow moves from left to right, the key distinction involves control over medical practice. Based on Porter's reasoning, this is the crucial variable for producing superior value and a competitive advantage in the marketplace.

Figure 5–3.   Control over Medical Practice in Managed Care Systems

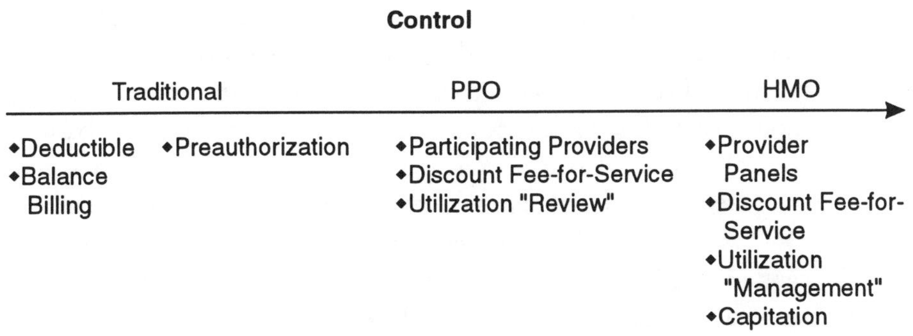

Control

Traditional		PPO	HMO
◆Deductible	◆Preauthorization	◆Participating Providers	◆Provider
◆Balance		◆Discount Fee-for-Service	Panels
Billing		◆Utilization "Review"	◆Discount Fee-for-Service
			◆Utilization "Management"
			◆Capitation

On the left, traditional indemnity health insurance has virtually no control over medical practice. Since members have complete freedom of choice, the only controls with this managed care arrangement are deductibles, balance billing, and preauthorization (which members have to implement). Under these circumstances, health costs have continued to escalate, as have premiums. Consequently, this system possesses the least inherent capacity to produce superior value.

PPOs are midway on the continuum. While the insurer uses financial incentives to steer members to preferred providers, the insurer and preferred provider are entirely separate institutionally. With PPOs, the insurer controls medical practice *indirectly*, through participating agreements with preferred providers. Because of this indirect control, many of the same conditions that led to inflation in medicine under more traditional circumstances operate under PPOs as well. PPOs, then, produce greater value compared to simpler systems of managed care, but their capacity to produce superior value is also limited.

On the right are HMOs. Unlike PPOs, HMOs try to exercise *direct* control over medical practice because they *both insure and deliver medical services*. In addition, since HMO members only receive coverage if they use HMO providers, all medical services fall within management's span of control. However, while HMOs have the potential to produce superior value, two structural tendencies endemic to their development have prevented that potential from being realized:

- ❏ First, as discussed earlier, there are many different HMO variations. These include direct contact arrangements, IPAs, PHOs, gatekeeper arrangements, salaried group models, and staff models. Even though all are technically HMOs, only the staff and salaried group model HMOs are formally organized to maintain *direct* control over medical practice. IPA, PHO, gatekeeper, and all other models are organized more like PPOs, in that participating agreements form the basis of control as opposed to direct management and supervision. That is, with the exception of HMOs in which physicians are salaried, virtually all HMOs contract with providers. Further, despite the trend towards capitating primary care physicians, most physician services in HMOs are still reimbursed as they would be under PPOs: On a discount fee-for-service basis. In other words, *the same piece-rate logic of produc-*

tivity associated with traditional health insurance also operates in the great majority of HMOs.

❑ Second, while HMOs, in theory, insure and deliver medical services, as a practical matter the pattern in HMO industry evolution has been for the *insurance and medical service functions to split off and assume relatively autonomous positions.*[31] The insurance position has become a "health plan," addressing such corporate roles as product design, finance, actuarial services, legal and regulatory activities, marketing, and information management. The medical service position has become the "provider arrangement," organized as IPA, PHO, or other non staff-model approaches. One marketing implication is that the health plan can offer a variety of product options, from strict HMO benefit designs to more flexible out-of-panel HMO, point-of-service, and PPO options. However, a second but far more significant strategic implication is that *HMOs' inherent capacity to directly control medical delivery has been severed from its insurance function. To achieve cost containment, HMOs have reverted to extracting discounts in the clinical process rather than producing greater value.*

Notwithstanding all the talk of a "managed care revolution," therefore, what bears emphasizing is that, for the great majority of HMOs, backward integration has not occurred. The structural relationship between HMOs as "buyers" and physician/hospital "suppliers" has not changed all that much from the more traditional health insurance-provider relationships that emerged after 1945. What has changed, of course, is a shift from the comfortable and smooth buyer-supplier relationships that existed up to even the early 1980s to the far more antagonistic relationships that exist today. I believe the deep-seated frustration physicians feel with managed care and the widespread recognition in policy circles that rationing in some form has to exist are both manifestations of HMOs in particular using the insurance industry's bargaining power to extract discounts from providers rather than pursue new forms of integration to produce greater value.

Clearly, part of the difficulty confronting HMO industry strategy is political. Physicians have always fiercely defended their professional autonomy

---

[31]Again, the two variations in which this argument does not apply are staff and salaried group model HMOs.

and the private practice model that goes with it. Consequently, the easiest and surest way for HMOs to achieve market entry has been to sign up physicians, rather than hire them. In addition, since mainstream America has never been oriented to "clinic" medicine, HMOs have tried to preserve the "look and feel" of private practice to assuage popular concerns about quality. Participating provider HMO arrangements, then, are typically easier to establish than staff or salaried group models. They also require far less capitalization. But HMO industry evolution is well beyond the introductory stage where market entry and consumer acceptance are at issue. Now that managed care is more advanced, what is at issue is how HMOs, along with PPOs and other managed care variations, use their different capabilities to meet the challenge of providing quality medicine before costs becomes prohibitive.

For their part, *HMOs have to determine whether they are paying for and producing medical services or just paying for medical services. If they are only paying, in my judgment they are not functioning as HMOs.* This is not a question of right or wrong. It is a question of strategy and structure. By paying for but not producing medical services, they have made a strategic decision to purchase but *not be in the business of directly organizing* the delivery of patient care. From Porter's standpoint, that decision formally shifts where the strategic focus should be in the value chain, as well as which value activities should be emphasized. Not recognizing this has the very real potential of putting HMOs at a competitive disadvantage; writ large, I believe it diminishes HMO industry performance overall.

Continuing along this same line, an HMO's decision not to produce medical services can still involve a strategy that relies on no out-of-panel coverage. But these managed care systems would then be structured as EPOs, not HMOs. As EPOs, there is no pretext that managed care actually controls how medical services are provided. Consequently, *operations*, as Porter defines it, "transforming inputs into final product form," assumes far less strategic significance in the total value chain compared to other value activities such as inbound logistics, outbound logistics, marketing and sales, and service.[32]

---

[32]Clearly, there are operational aspects in all five value activities, but "operations" in Porter's scheme refers to that aspect of the total business system in which the *production process* literally occurs. For this reason, operations herein refers to *medical practice*.

Consider, now, two nonstaff-model HMOs competing in the same market: One redefines itself as an EPO; the other continues as an HMO. Senior management in the EPO decides that its key value activities are *marketing and sales*, and *inbound logistics*. The marketing and sales emphasis addresses benefit design and the provider network. For benefit design, management establishes deductibles and co-payments to price their product extremely low. For the provider panel, the commitment is to have both a large number and the most respected primary care physicians, with a much narrower band of specialists linked to center of excellence relationships. The EPO's second major emphasis is inbound logistics. Here, resources are devoted to building an electronic and cashless environment so that members use their credit card at the provider's office, and have the wherewithall to go out-of-panel whenever they chose. At the end of the month, members receive simple monthly statements with a variety of payment options. In addition, the system's point-of-sale capability captures clinical data for management reporting purposes. Thus, the EPO's whole approach to utilization review is revamped. Panel members are routinely profiled and compared to peer norms, but the false premise of "managing care" no longer applies. Also, while physicians are not happy with the EPO's fee schedule, they are pleased to be paid in a timely fashion.

The EPO's competitor, on the other hand, continues to position itself as an "HMO." By default, *operations* becomes the main value activity in the organization's value chain. Since it is not a staff or salaried group model HMO, management has little choice but to rely heavily on utilization management to control inputs. This emphasis generates more headaches than it's worth. No matter what management does, no matter where it squeezes, no matter how much software or how many employees are thrown at the process, no matter how rigorous the provider report card, medical practice cannot be controlled, and costs do not go down. Compounding these operational difficulties is a growing resentment among physicians as well as patients. Physicians complain about devoting more energy to bureaucratic matters than medicine, about losing control over how they treat their patients, and about withholds and per-member per-month (pmpm) payments that cause them to actually lose money. For their part, patients complain about being treated like "cattle" in their physician's office and about the quality of the physician panel.

In comparing the two competitors, the EPO clearly did not produce value *in the clinical process*. But the HMO did not either. The EPO did, though, produce value through the two activities in the value chain that management chose to emphasize: Marketing and sales, and inbound logistics. Unlike the HMO, the EPO succeeded where it concentrated its resources. Indeed, the more the HMO concentrated on operations, the more efficiency decreased along with customer satisfaction. To hold members' out-of-pocket costs down, the HMO was eventually forced to increase premiums, while the EPO's already low premiums held constant. Despite the EPO starting off on shaky ground, it gradually attracted growing employer interest. Conversely, the HMO's competitive position deteriorated.

This case illustrates a number of strategic lessons that build on the application of Porter's value chain to managed care:[33]

Lesson # 1. All managed care systems are business systems encompassing five core functions or value activities. These value activities comprise the value chain. Each of the five value activities in a managed care business system produces an entirely different kind of value. Figure 5–4 is an adaptation of Porter's value chain to a generic managed care system, be it HMO or PPO. My suggestion for which functions and tasks conform to which value activity in the value chain are shown below.

Significantly, *operations focuses solely on the production of clinical value*. Other value activities may influence the production of clinical value, but for all intents and purposes they have nothing to do with producing clinical value. They produce different kinds of value. One of the most important strategic questions that senior management in any managed care system has to answer is to what degree operations can produce clinical value. Since it is physician decision making that dictates diagnosis and treatment, operations in managed care depends on how effectively it can control physician performance. *If physician performance cannot be controlled, and controlled effectively, it might well be that this value activity should not be a high priority*—in which case, management should ask what other value activity or activities should be a priority? As the case above demonstrated, competitive premi-

---

[33]These lessons are developed much more extensively in Chapter 6.

Figure 5–4.   Value Production in Managed Care Systems

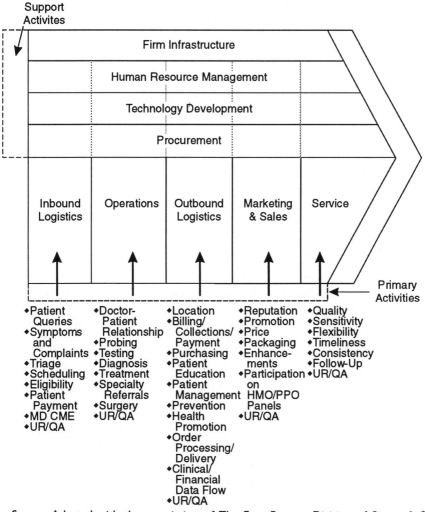

Support
Activites

| Firm Infrastructure |
| Human Resource Management |
| Technology Development |
| Procurement |

| Inbound Logistics | Operations | Outbound Logistics | Marketing & Sales | Service |

Primary Activities

◆Patient Queries
◆Symptoms and Complaints
◆Triage
◆Scheduling
◆Eligibility
◆Patient Payment
◆MD CME
◆UR/QA

◆Doctor-Patient Relationship
◆Probing
◆Testing
◆Diagnosis
◆Treatment
◆Specialty Referrals
◆Surgery
◆UR/QA

◆Location
◆Billing/ Collections/ Payment
◆Purchasing
◆Patient Education
◆Patient Management
◆Prevention
◆Health Promotion
◆Order Processing/ Delivery
◆Clinical/ Financial Data Flow
◆UR/QA

◆Reputation
◆Promotion
◆Price
◆Packaging
◆Enhance-ments
◆Participation on HMO/PPO Panels
◆UR/QA

◆Quality
◆Sensitivity
◆Flexibility
◆Timeliness
◆Consistency
◆Follow-Up
◆UR/QA

Source: Adapted with the permission of The Free Press, a Division of Simon & Schuster from *Competitive Advantage: Creating and Sustaining Superior Performance* by Michael E. Porter. Copyright © 1985 by Michael E. Porter.

ums are not necessarily dependent on the management of medical inputs; other value activities can also play a key role.

Lesson # 2. Given that HMOs, alone among managed care systems, both pay for and deliver medical services, *operations has to be the critical value activity in an HMO's value chain.* If operations is not a strong and effective value activity, HMOs should either strengthen that capacity or cease being

HMOs. The key variable is whether HMO operations is in a position to directly control medical practice. Because direct control only emanates from staff or salaried situations, all contractually based HMOs have an inherent weakness in that they have to impose external controls (utilization review/utilization management) on independent physicians in private practice. The more HMOs depend on external controls, the more two forms of inefficiency crop up: 1) alienating physicians, the very producers they (and patients) depend on; and 2) stimulating churning and other attempts by physicians to game the system. With the majority of HMOs in the United States organized around participating providers, managed care in general, I believe, would be better served if such HMOs either evolve to staff or salaried group models or redefine themselves as EPOs, POS, plans and PPOs.

Lesson # 3. There is an enormous difference between "consolidation" and "integration" in healthcare industry evolution, and one should not be confused with the other. Where consolidation is external to a business system's value chain, integration is internal. Consolidation involves reducing duplicate functions, spreading fixed costs, merging with competitors, and gaining market share. Consolidation may well be necessary for integration but in and of itself does not constitute integration. Integration entails linkages between value activities that bear on production and distribution, such as altering the division of labor or infusing more advanced forms of technology into the work process. Integration can be between any two value activities in the value chain; or it can be vertical, between a value chain and the value activities of its buyers and/or suppliers. A basic challenge HMOs, PPOs, and other managed care systems face today is to *achieve more effective integration inside their value chains, as well as between their value chains and the value activities of providers on the one hand and patients on the other.*

Lesson # 4. With HMOs today offering deductibles, co-payments and out-of-panel coverage, and PPOs offering EPO products, the key difference between managed care systems is not in benefit design or closed versus open panels. The key difference is in the *kind of integration a managed care system makes possible and the kind of value such integration helps to produce.* It is here that staff and salaried group-model HMOs stand apart from all other managed care arrangements because integration in their value chain can extend to operations and the production of clinical value. The same cannot be said for any contractually based HMO, EPO, PPO, or POS plan. Management in none of these arrangements has the prerogative to either rework the clinical division of labor or redefine how technology is incorporated in the clinical process.

Lesson # 5. Ultimately, *managed care systems are organized around one of two axial principles: They either produce healthcare services, or they purchase healthcare from others who are the producers.* Consequently, there really are only two basic kinds of managed care systems: Staff and salaried group-model systems and contractually-based systems. From a management standpoint, this lesson has two strategic implications:

❑ First, managed care systems should clearly adopt one of these two axial principles and then position themselves accordingly. Failing to do so, puts them, in Porter's words, "stuck in the middle"—trying to produce and purchase healthcare services through mechanisms that confound doing either.

❑ Second, managed care systems should evaluate their more significant design features (e.g., reimbursement methodologies, network strategy, utilization management techniques) by how effectively they lend themselves to either of the two axial principles: Producing or purchasing health services.

From the standpoint of strategy, managed care systems can be divided into two camps: Those that can directly control medical inputs and those that cannot. In the first camp, the focus should be on *producing clinical value* and then developing linkages from operations to other value activities. In the second camp, the focus should be on *purchasing* and developing linkages primarily through nonoperations value activities to produce other kinds of value. To the extent the "staff or salaried group-model camp" avoids concentrating first and foremost on the production of clinical value, it neglects both a powerful source of competitive advantage and an opportunity to improve the quality of health services that managed care offers. To the extent the "contractually based camp" persists in trying to produce clinical value, it will continue alienating providers, neglecting value activities that could make various nonclinical aspects of managed care both more integral and attractive to the public as a whole.

CHAPTER 6

Strategy in the Information Age

The dichotomy between medicine's enormous clinical potential and the system's inability to control healthcare expenditures represents one of the most compelling contradictions in our society today. The capacity to sustain investments in basic and applied research, to afford public and private sector health insurance, and to deliver quality healthcare equitably have all been threatened. Curiously, those in government and private industry find themselves in a situation not unlike the one Jack Kent Cooke was in some years ago when as the owner of the Washington Redskins he was forced to justify firing his popular coach, the late George Allen. Cooke's explanation: "I gave him an unlimited budget and he exceeded it."[1] Similarly, despite all the efforts of corporate benefit managers, insurance industry executives, and government leaders to rein in the rising cost of healthcare, the system continues to exceed its unlimited budget.

---

[1] Cited in Donald Cohodes. "The Loss of Innocence," *Healthcare and Its Costs.* Carl Schramm, ed. (New York: Norton, 1987), 83.

In past chapters, I have used insights from leading business strategists to suggest that at least part of the problem can be traced to the misapplication of strategy to current healthcare industry circumstances. In this chapter, I want to suggest that part of the problem can also be traced to changing industry circumstances.

The circumstances I'm referring to derive from what is now widely viewed as the "post-industrial" or "information age" economy in the U.S. Stanley Davis' *Future Perfect*, and a second volume he coauthored with Bill Davidson, *2020 Vision*, delve into the nature and behavior of this economy[2] The two volumes depict basic changes confronting business and industry today, changes that call for a sea change in strategic thinking. In *Future Perfect*, Davis writes, "Einstein said new frameworks are like climbing a mountain—the larger view encompasses, rather than rejects, the earlier, more restricted view" (1987, 194–195). To their credit, both texts point to a larger, more encompassing view for business strategy in general–a view I hope to show has great merit for business strategy in medicine as well.

MODELS

With a single stroke, Davis neatly summarizes a series of relationships extending from the history of science to the history of business, relationships that highlight the difficulties current business strategy confronts in the information age:

> It is no accident that Sir Isaac Newton came before Adam Smith, whose theories in turn had to be spelled out before Henry Ford could create the assembly line and Alfred Sloan could then devise the divisional corporate structure. A basic progression governs the evolution of management in all market economies: Fundamental properties of the *universe* are transformed into *scientific* under-

---

2 Stanley M. Davis. *Future Perfect* (New York: Addison-Wesley, 1987) © 1987 by Stanley M. Davis. Reprinted by permission of Addison-Wesley Publishing Company, Inc.; and Stan Davis and Bill Davidson. *2020 Vision: Transform Your Business Today To Succeed in Tomorrow's Economy* (New York: Simon and Schuster, 1991) Copyright © 1991 by William H. Davidson and Stanley M. Davis. Reprinted by permission of Simon & Schuster, Inc. This chapter is focused on Stan Davis because most of the discussion draws upon his work, *Future Perfect*. Wherever *2020 Vision* is used, I will refer to both Davis and Davidson.

standing, then developed into new *technologies*, which are applied to create new products and services for *business*, which then ultimately define our models of *organization*.

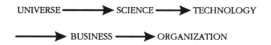

The dilemma for managers is that dominant organization models are the last link in the progression to develop, and are not likely to occur until the economy is fairly mature. While the new economy is in the early decades of its unfolding, businesses continue to use organization models that were more appropriate to previous times than to current needs (1987, 5).

What Davis' comments suggest about business organization today is that *we have industrial models of organization driving a post-industrial economy* (1987, 6). The terms "industrial" and "post-industrial," though, should not imply that economic eras are mutually exclusive. Industrial manufacturing is no less vital to today's economy than agriculture was when manufacturing put its stamp on agrarian society years ago. But the relationship between industrial production and information systems has changed. In the same way we would not impose an agrarian logic on an industrial economy, we should not impose an industrial logic on a post-industrial economy. We need to change our approach to business strategy if we are to master the opportunities inherent in the information age.

Insofar as strategic thinking lags behind the scientific and technological foundation of the information age, mediocrity is the big winner. From the standpoint of the marketplace, the implication is that marginal improvements are simply not enough to succeed. "You can get 5, 10, 15 percent improvements in what you are doing by doing the same thing, only a bit better," Davis and Davidson argue. If competitors have reworked their business to be more in tune with the capabilities of the information age, however, their improvement may well be in multiples of 100, 300, or 500 percent. Industrially framed businesses in a post-industrial world can't just do things better than their competitors and hope to have a realistic chance for success. They have to do things in a fundamentally different way and, in the process, transform their business (1991, 15).

Davis and Davidson cite as one example, the transformation of the bathroom fixture business in Japan:

> Japan's leading fixture manufacturer, Toto Ltd., now sells a "paperless" toilet that sprays warm water like a bidet, blows warm air to dry, and even dispenses a scent. "Smart" toilet/bidets are now common in Japan. The machine keeps the seat warm in winter and automatically sanitizes the bowl after each use. In other words, you can control the water pressure, temperature and angle of the spray. New models analyze urine and measure body temperature, weight, blood pressure and pulse. More than five million smart units have been sold, and the product is just being introduced into the American market. Bathroom fixtures is a very mature business that has found new growth from the introduction of information into the ceramic core of its products. We are in the age of smart toilets (1991, 15–16).

"Smart toilets" highlight an important principle for business strategy: In every economy, it is the core technology that propels growth and development. In today's economy, this means that for businesses just starting up, those wanting to expand, or those needing to revitalize, the requirement is the same: *Informationalize.* "From small mom-and-pop stores to giant global corporations, the point to grasp is not merely that all economic activities will depend upon information to create and control their destiny. . . . The point is that economic value from generating, using and selling information is growing significantly faster than the value added by producing traditional goods and services." *It is not the production of goods and services that is the critical factor for success; it is the production of information content in goods and services.* "Increasing the information content of any product or service, to make a smart version of a not-so-smart one," is now the basis for competitive advantage. "All businesses will get increasingly smart, in this sense, or yield to more informationalized competitors" (1991, 17).

VALUE

While every economy produces value, not all value is the same or equal. There is a hierarchy of values. Though Davis did not develop his argument in just this way, I would hazard the following hypothesis about the evolution and hierarchy of economic value. Value in all economies is mediated by supply/demand relationships and *the* underlying production standard presupposed in the technology of the time. In hunting and gathering economies, *need* was the underlying production standard; in agrarian economies, it was *difficulty*, in industrial economies, it is *production time*; and in post-industrial economies, what Davis calls *"any time"* is the underlying production standard. These relationships are depicted in Figure 6–1.

Figure 6–1.   Production of Value in Economic Evolution

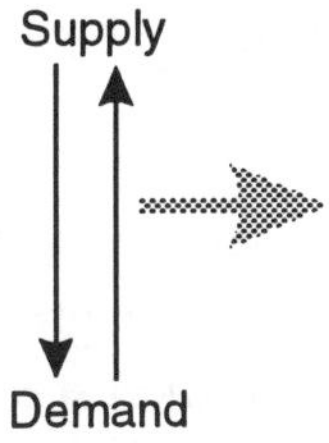

Supply

Production Standard   Economy

Need . . . . Hunting and Gathering
Difficulty . . . . Agrarian
Production Time . . . . Industrial
Any Time . . . . Post-Industrial

Demand

Possibly the most difficult thing to understand about value is that at its core it is perceptual in nature. How we choose to understand value tells us a lot about how we view its production. Currently, according to Davis, value is understood primarily from the producer's perspective. Costs of production. Reliance on inputs. The making of something. Instead, he argues, value should be understood from the *consumer's perspective*. An industrial perspective defines value by what goes on in the production process up to the actual consumer. A post-industrial perspective defines value at the point of consumption per se. "The transformative quality lies in the elimination of any waiting time at all—'zero-based time.' Whenever the customer needs a product or service offered, it should be immediately available. . . . We are talking about instantaneous products and services . . . truly a holistic conception of the product" (1987, 15).

Davis lists three principles that operate under this *any time standard of value*:

❑ "Consumers need products and services ANY TIME (i.e., in their time frame, not the providers')."

❑ "Producers who deliver their products and services in REAL TIME, relative to their competitors, will have a decided advantage."

❑ "Operating in real time means no LAG TIME between identification and fulfillment of the need" (1987, 16).

What are the strategic implications of this argument? First, "whatever your business, think about how you can create products and services in real time that you can deliver instantly" (1987, 15). This does not mean it can always be done, or that it can always be done completely. But it is *a standard that business in post-industrial economies should strive for.* The closer a business approaches production according to the "any time" standard, the more value it produces. Business "gains competitive advantage simply by being able to move from identifying to satisfying market needs faster than one's competitors—faster than the 'industry' leader and/or the 'industry' average" (1987, 19).

Second, management's task is to analyze the value chain at every point and determine where approaching the any time standard would have the greatest impact on the overall business. "If A and B are linked together, then specific inputs to A should alter B almost simultaneously. In earlier technologies there were time lags between events A and B. Electronics introduced the real-time world of almost no time lags. . . . But while today's technologies operate in real time, today's organizations do not." Managers in the post-industrial economy need to find ways to reduce the constraints their organization places on technology, that is, make the necessary changes in organization to "reduce the time lags between inputs and outcomes" (1987, 19, 23).

Finally, the approach that strategic thinking takes toward the present needs to change. In industrial models, Davis suggests, business operates in three spatial dimensions: 1) span of control; 2) hierarchy; and 3) geographic territory (1987, 41). Post-industrial economies add a fourth dimension: time. The introduction of this fourth dimension, he argues, "is akin to shifting from a Newtonian sense of time as an absolute to an Einsteinian sense of time's relativity. . . . The sense of time that executives employ with the industrial model is to use the present organization as the vehicle for getting to the future" (1987, 25). The sense of time Davis insists executives should employ in a post-industrial context "is to *lead from a place in time that assumes you are already there, and that is determined even though it hasn't happened yet*" (1987, 25). He draws on the sociologist Alfred Schutz, to highlight this point:

The actor projects this action as if it were already over and done with and lying in the past. . . . Strangely enough, therefore, because it is pictured as completed, the planned act bears the temporal character of pastness. . . . The fact that it was thus pictured as if it were simultaneously past and future can be taken care of by saying that it is thought of in the future-perfect sense.[3]

In post-industrial economies, producing superior value requires that strategic thinking be conducted in the "future-perfect" sense. That means planning and managing for a reality which has yet to occur—like arriving on a supersonic plane and preparing for passengers on a regular flight who have yet to arrive (Davis, 38). It also means building future goals and objectives into current directives and actions so the future flows almost intuitively from the present. *Where strategy in an industrial context tries to make the present into the future, strategy in a post-industrial context tries to shape the present by the future.* Quoting Harold Geneen, Davis sums up his approach to strategic thinking thusly: "You read a book from the beginning to the end. You run a business the opposite way. You start with the end, and then do everything you must to reach it" (1987, 28).

Davis and Davidson expand on this last principle by distinguishing between business and organization. "A *business* applies resources to create products and services that meet market needs. . . . An *organization* is the way those resources are administered—the housekeeping—which includes the structure, systems, employees and culture of the organization." The present organization, they argue, is generally a poor indicator of what is needed for the future. "Since you should organize in relation to the kind of business you will be in, that not-yet-existing business is the best source of information for what the future organization should look like." The strategist's responsibility is to get a good fix on the future business, understand the organization it will require, and shape the present organization so it can serve the future business. *The best place to look for your current strategy is in your future business; the worst place is in your current organization* (1991, 112–113).

---

3 Schutz, quoted in Davis, 26. Schutz's statement was drawn from Karl Weick. *The Social Psychology of Organizing* (Reading, MA: Addison-Wesley, 1969). No page reference was indicated.

SPACE

Miniaturization is a key feature of post-industrial economies. "The new technologies, built around lasers, fiber optics, genetic engineering, silicon and artificial intelligence all pack more micromatter into less micro space than did the industrial technologies" (1987, 44). Miniaturization allows information to travel faster, improve product reliability, and reduce costs. Miniaturization also bears on the production of value in that it allows products and services to provide either the same capabilities in less space, or additional capabilities in the same space. "Miniaturize something enough," Davis suggests, "and space becomes more of a resource and less of a constraint" (1987, 45–48).

For Davis, perhaps the most important implication of miniaturization is that it pushes *production capability into the physical space of the consumer*, enabling the consumer to literally take over at least some of the producer's actions in their own space (1987, 54). As examples, Davis cites home banking and computer aided design, which lets customers design their own products according to their own specifications. In different degrees, the latter is now surfacing in the clothing, hair dressing, home construction, and automobile industries.[4] It is also evident in home healthcare, and could well become prominent in other aspects of healthcare as well. There are two practical messages here. The first is that consumers are more likely to purchase products they can have with them wherever they are, rather than purchase competing products. The second is that *business strategy in post-industrial economies should focus on moving the production process down the value chain to distribution and sales in order to be as close to the customer as possible* (1987, 53–55).

In the same way that the producer's space is moving into physical space of the consumer, the functions that occur in the space between producer and consumer are changing. Be it corporations, public administration, manufacturing, or marketing, one of the distinguishing characteristics of industrial economies is the enormous amount of space that intermediation takes up between the producer of goods and services and the end consumer. According to the inner logic of industrial economies, the more intermediation there is in the value

---

4 For clothing see Glen Rifkin. "Digital Blue Jeans Pour Data and Legs Into Customized Fit." *New York Times* (November 11, 1994): A1.

chain, the more value is produced. According to the inner logic of post-industrial economies, intermediation adds inefficiency and costs that are passed on to the consumer and ultimately borne by society. *Disintermediation, therefore, should be one of the main objectives of business strategy in postindustrial economies* (1987, 60–61).

The need to rethink strategy toward space is particularly important for business in post-industrial economies. Hierarchy is the foundation of industrial organization. The reasons can be traced to the imperatives of knowledge, coordination, and control in the organization of industrial economies. In post-industrial economies, however, these imperatives are diminished because information can be linked throughout the value chain in what Davis calls "any time, any place." Expert systems giving generalists the knowledge of specialists, information networks bringing necessary knowledge to one's finger tips instantly, computer aided design reducing the number of steps that are required between initial concept and final product, and simulation capabilities that simplify operational planning, all diminish the imperatives for hierarchy in organization. As post-industrial economies unfold, hierarchy in organizations should lessen, Davis points out, not because of a shift in values, but because of the transformative power that information technologies bring to business. *If you want to peer into the future shape of post-industrial organizations, "look to the constraints of time, place and mass" that are reduced by information age technologies* (1987, 79–83).

INTANGIBLE VERSUS TANGIBLE

When dividing the whole into its parts, it is the space between the parts that unites them into a single whole. Space is intangible, but what should be understood about post-industrial economies is that as information embedded in the parts increases, the parts become increasingly intangible as well (1987, 77). If you were to analyze the total economic pie in post-industrial economies, more and more of the value produced and consumed could be defined as intangible as opposed to tangible. The growth in the proportion of what is intangibile over what is tangible can be traced to information-based technologies making space between the parts of the whole as productive, if not more productive, than the parts themselves. This is because 1) information is "de-materializing" what matters most; 2) information is the source for a growing proportion of value produced; and 3) information linkages are the critical determinant of efficiency and competitive advantage in the marketplace. *Part of the changing mindset management requires in post-industrial economies is that strategy should focus on the relationships that unite the whole, rather than on either the parts themselves or the relationships between the parts.* Davis and Davidson amplify this point with the comment that it used to be if you built a better mousetrap, the world beat a path to your door; whereas, now you have to build a better path (1991, 59–60).

These developments point to basic changes in the inner workings of market forces themselves. In post-industrial economies, informationalized relationships and "infostructure" drive business performance by determining not only with whom you can link and therefore to whom you can sell, but also how much those linkages are worth. Value-added in this context can accrue not only to the end customer, as we ordinarily think, but also to the producer because electronic linkages dramatically expand the producer's ability to learn from and feed back the consumer's knowledge into the original producer's operation. This marks a dramatic change from the relationship between market share and experience in industrial economies described in the Henderson chapter. Where industrial economies presupposed relationships of *output* and efficiency, post-industrial economies presuppose relationships of *outcomes* and efficiency. The change is extremely significant because it holds out the prospect of genuine progress in the quality of life produced by post-industrial economies, progress that can be seen in three ways: 1) efficiency throughout the value chain can now result from outcomes instead of simply outputs; 2) lower-volume producers can achieve the same efficiency as higher-volume producers; and 3) qualitative standards can be elevated over quantitative ones in the indicators governing economic performance.[5]

---

[5] For an excellent example of qualitative considerations driving quantitative ones in standards of manufacturing performance, see James P. Womack, Daniel T. Jones, and Daniel Roos. *The Machine That Changed The World: The Story of Lean Production* (New York: Harper Collins, 1991). "Lean production," the method of manufacturing that Toyota pioneered, is distinguished from "mass production," which Henry Ford pioneered. The former is entirely focused on quality considerations in the production process; the latter, on quantitative considerations. In a somewhat different context, Davis also distinguishes between output and outcomes. He cites as references Michael B. Packer. "Measuring the Intangible in Productivity." *Technology Review* (February–March 1983); and Robert S. Kaplan. "Yesterday's Accounting Undermines Production." *Harvard Business Review* (July–August 1984).

Davis ties these developments to three separate observations about management in the post-industrial era. First, since tangible products and services will produce less and less value, and intangible products and services will produce more, capital should be invested increasingly in intangible capabilities and proportionately less in tangible ones. *"The degree to which a business can increase its products' i/t ratios faster than the competition's is an important competitive advantage"* (1987, 113, italics added). Davis reinforces this point by quoting the economist Paul Hawken who argued that: "The single most important trend to understand is the changing ratio between mass and information in goods and services" (1987, 101).[6]

Second, knowing whether intangibles are at the core or at the periphery of a business is central to strategic thinking in post-industrial economies. *Managers who consciously work with the intangible aspects of their business will push ahead of their tangible-oriented competitors* (1987, 94). This requires: 1) changing accounting practices so the information and service components of tangible products can be captured; 2) rethinking what is core and peripheral to the basic business; and 3) visualizing intangible approaches and outlets for tangible products and services. It also requires a much more intense focus on informationalization throughout the value chain. According to Davis and Davidson, "Firms that establish informationalized operations and relationships in any business will gain a significant edge because they provide much greater precision in ordering to exact specifications, shorter response times, working capital savings, and significant overhead reductions" (1991, 72).

Finally, drawing on the noted business historian Alfred Chandler and his Pulitzer Prize winning book, *The Visible Hand*, Davis makes the point that with the transition from an industrial to a post-industrial economy senior decision makers need to manage business "context" more and "content" less. The emphasis in the early industrial era was on the external forces of the market, or the "invisible hand" Adam Smith referred to; whereas, the latter industrial era emphasized internal forces of management, or the "visible hand" Chandler refers to. Management's main challenge now, according to Davis, is contextual: While we are shifting from the tangible and visible hand of an industrial economy to the intangible and invisible hand of a

---

6 Paul Hawken. *The Next Economy* (New York: Holt, Rinehart & Winston, 1983), 11.

post-industrial economy, post-industrial organization has not shifted commensurately (1987, 109–110). Strategically, what this means is that business leaders have to redesign their organizations so that the thrust of today's business can be directed to: 1) the intangible value information technology produces; 2) the embeddedness of knowledge in relationships between production and consumption; and 3) the potential for production to migrate more closely to the end consumer.

It should be reemphasized that Davis' view of strategy is not that industrialization and manufacturing are irrelevant and information-age technology is all-important. His point is that their role in the scheme of things has changed. The Rosetta stone for business strategy now resides in the possibilities presupposed in a post-industrial economy. This suggests that information and intangibility are at the center of what is required to build and maintain a competitive advantage and that they should be leveraged, first to stretch the high-tech horizon outward, and second to improve all lesser means of production that continue to be necessary for society in post-industrial economies.

A NOTE ON THE RENAISSANCE AND THE INFORMATION AGE

One of the most significant developments in the history of medicine was a transition that occurred some five centuries ago from medical thought organized around high theory to medical thought organized around empirical science. For over 1,500 years prior to the Renaissance, Western medicine was based on ancient Greek and Roman clinical observations tied to medieval Christian belief. That doctrine centered on concepts of disease and treatment which upheld the Church's teachings on sin and spirituality as well as the individual's place in the great "chain of being." With the Renaissance, an entire worldview linking the Church and medicine began to give way. An important catalyst in this transition was the growing legitimacy of a surgical perspective in medical training. Where barber-surgeons had a much lower status than physician-clerics throughout the Middle Ages, the Renaissance set into motion a series of developments that elevated the status surgery. These developments revolved around the empirical study of human anatomy and physiology. While medicine from the 16th through the 19th centuries continued to do more harm than good in patient care, the great breakthroughs from Harvey to Virchow that form the bedrock of modern medical science have their origins in the surgical thinking initiated by the Renaissance. Do the information-age capabilities of a post-industrial economy pose analogous possibilities *for modern medical organization* today? That question is depicted in Figure 6–2.

Figure 6–2.   The Renaissance and the Information Age

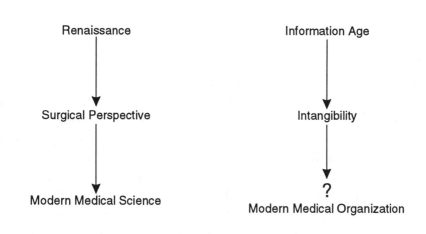

Davis' work suggests the answer *could be* yes. Indeed, it might well be that the possibilities offered by a post-industrial economy represent the critical yardstick for determining where organizational developments in the health-care industry can catch up with the clinical achievements of medical science. A lot depends on whether opportunities are seized, on whether capabilities are half-heartedly or more systematically used, and on whether key decision makers have the willingness to change. A lot also depends on the kind of strategic thinking those decision makers draw on. This last issue will be the focus of the remainder of the chapter.

POST-INDUSTRIAL MANAGED CARE STRATEGY

In past chapters, I argued that an underlying goal of managed competition is to industrialize an industry that was never industrialized. My point was that physicians have enjoyed a degree of independence and autonomy inconsistent with the interests of cost containment. To counter physician independence, managed competition promotes the growth of market forces to impose a discipline on the professional role comparable to the discipline industrialization imposed on craft production. The point I would make now, however, is that *managed care's frame of reference should not be industrial. We need to post-industrialize medicine, not industrialize it.* The following is a preliminary sketch of just some of the major elements that might be considered in post-industrial strategic thinking for medicine under for managed care.

Element # 1: Develop a Post-Industrial Production Mentality

A critical message in Davis' work is that *when the technological capabilities of an economy are constrained by organization in business, less and less value is produced relative to the needs of society.* The value problem Davis poses could be likened to the agrarian problem Malthus posed almost two centuries ago. The difference is that where Malthus assumed population growth would *naturally* exceed productive capacity, Davis assumes productive capacity can meet or even exceed a population's needs. For Davis, the issue turns on whether the productive capacity of an economy adequately draws on the technological means it has at its disposal. If not, then the needs society generates outstrip the value its economy produces. That's the mark of a society in decline, which might well be one of the core problems confronting the United States today.

This theme can be extended to business organization through Porter's work on the value chain and from Porter to the healthcare industry under managed care. Porter makes the point that the value chain is the basis for competitive advantage, that differences in particular value activities expose strengths and weaknesses on which competitive advantage is based, and that firms should manage such value activities by adopting initiatives which yield the greatest comparative advantage. Insofar as firms don't do this, they run the risk of losing out in one of four ways: 1) to competitors; 2) to substitute products; 3) to buyers and/or suppliers pursuing strategies of backward and/or forward integration, respectively; and 4) to deteriorating industry conditions. It's the latter, I believe, that characterizes much of the current healthcare industry.

In the broadest terms, I would account for the deterioration in industry conditions as follows:

1. The healthcare system suffers from a *value deficit*. This deficit is rooted in a contradiction between the demands placed on that system, and the system's inability to produce the value needed to meet such demands. The demands themselves are secular in nature. Whether due to a growth in clinical intensity or in acuity as a result of aging, AIDS, cancer, and a host of other chronic and degenerative diseases, secular pressures are an invariant force in the healthcare system. At the same time, the system, with all of the managed care that has been brought to bear, has not controlled the inflationary spiral caused by these pressures.[7] Since neither government, insurers, nor employers can afford a continuation of the recent pattern of healthcare inflation, managed care has turned to various *rationing* approaches as a way of controlling costs. These approaches include benefit limitations, gatekeeper provisions, global budgets, capitation, and other forms of prospective reimbursement.

2. Rationing focuses on reducing the demands placed on the healthcare system rather than improving the productive capacity to meet such demands. It targets patients on the one hand and providers, most notably physicians (supply-induced demand), on the other. Its purpose is to constrain both the intensity and velocity of service activity as well as the dollar amounts actually paid for said services. This Malthusian bias is fundamentally at odds with the goals of modern medical science. That managed care in its current form is an intellectual descendent of Malthus bears special emphasis. For Malthus, as for managed care right now, a central tenant involves limits: Limits in agricultural production or limits in an

---

7 See, for example, the General Accounting Office Report, *Managed Healthcare Effect on Employers' Costs Difficult to Measure*, GAO/HRD-94-3 (October, 1993); Robert Pear. "Medicare to Stop Pushing Patients to HMOs: Idea Fails to Save Money." *New York Times* (December 27, 1993): A1; and Jerry Geisel. "Nation's Healthcare Bill to Top $1 Trillion in 1994." *Business Insurance* (January 3, 1994): 2. Geisel sites a U.S. Department of Commerce report estimating an increase in national healthcare expenditures of 12.5 percent from 1993 to 1994 as compared to a 12.1 percent increase from 1992 to 1993. The report estimated healthcare expenditures as a percentage of gross domestic product to be 15% in 1994, compared to 14 percent in 1993 and 13% in 1992. In addition, "The 12.5% rise in national healthcare expenditures forecast for 1994 is substantially greater than the 10.5% increase in 1987 . . . "

economy's ability to produce affordable healthcare. Malthus, of course, completely underestimated the productive capacity of an industrial economy to meet society's agricultural needs just as, in my judgment, managed care underestimates the productive capacity of a post-industrial economy to efficiently meet society's healthcare needs. Rather than managed care trying to improve production, it relies on rationing to limit production. By and large, this means applying brakes to a system that is desperate for cost containment. Such braking action is at the center of the deteriorating industry conditions in healthcare today.

3. Managed care's various rationing strategies lock physicians in the very same conditions that created the system's problems to begin with. This issue goes beyond resource limitations and involves the basic framework joining managed care systems to physicians. In effect, *the organization rationing generates arrests the development of newer, more productive forms of clinical capacity.* The following are some examples of how organizational relationships associated with managed care rationing impede progress toward new levels of practice development:

   ❑ **Shifting the Risk.** It has become axiomatic for payors, particularly HMOs, to shift the risk from those who control the dollars to those who provide the services. This was graphically illustrated in a recent meeting I had with the vice president of a major medical center who had the task of building an HMO for his institution. Because the medical center was both prominent and well capitalized, its move was taken seriously by local competitors. What surprised me was the way it was taken seriously. As word spread about its intentions, at least six HMOs approached the medical center to either buy their total operation outright or buy a substantial equity stake. These HMOs, all based on IPA, medical group, or PHO arrangements, had no confidence in their own ability to control rising costs and were looking for a way to, if not exit the industry, at least reduce their exposure. If HMOs are questioning their own ability to effectively control costs, then shifting the risk merely displaces functional problems that have yet to be adequately solved.

   ❑ **Shifting the Bureaucracy.** One of the great myths in managed care is that capitation eliminates administration. It doesn't. When HMOs shift their risk, they also shift layers of bureaucracy to capitated IPAs,

PHOs, and medical groups that take on many of the responsibilities HMOs regularly assume: Day-to-day administration, provider relations, MIS, internal claims processing, finance, utilization review, quality assurance, and monthly reporting. Capitation gives providers exclusivity over a patient population, something they dearly want. But in exchange for exclusivity, they become a mini-insurance operation—developing in-house what is typically called an MSO or management service organization. *This process immerses the physician organization in the details of insurance industry functions rather than the details of practice organization.* So long as physician energy, ingenuity and attention are directed in this fashion, the opportunity for physicians to develop more productive clinical capacity diminishes.[8]

❑ **Shell Strategies and Shock Treatment.** More than one physician has told me that practicing medicine under managed care is like being in the "twilight zone." Much of this I attribute to the shock treatment that follows from the overlay of capitated and heavily discounted arrangements on a fee-for-service environment. When HMOs capitate an IPA or PHO, for example, they put a managed care shell on physicians who continue to operate in a solo practice manner. The expectation is that a rigorous capitation will induce physicians to become more efficient. Aside from physicians being notoriously poor businesspeople and poor managers, though, the brute fact is that the fee-for-service environment contains absolute limits in the *kinds* of productivity gains physicians are capable of achieving.[9] The lack of integration among physicians, their lack of coordination, the absence of a single, well-honed division of labor, and the persistence of highly

---

8 As an alternative to reproducing mini-HMO operations by developing an MSO, IPAs, PHOs, and medical groups can contract with an outside MSO to provide the necessary claims processing, UR, and administrative services. Even under these circumstances, though, physician energy is still directed more towards coping with the insurance bureaucracy (now much more directly involved in their personal time and practice orbit) than finding innovative ways to make the practice of medicine more productive.

9 Instead of stimulating physician interest in clinical productivity, the tendency is for IPAs and PHOs to create more physician headaches: a) paperwork along with the pressure to justify tests, referrals, and surgery continues; b) provider is pitted against provider in the zero-sum world of capitation; and c) collegial perceptions are defined by performing under budget rather than how well one performs. In addition, *the capitation IPAs and PHOs receive from HMOs rarely, if ever, reflects the costs of administration.* As a result, the administrative capacity that physicians develop is usually poorly capitalized, resulting in a platform that satisfies minimum operational needs rather than promoting first-class operations.

individualistic practice orientations, all militate against efficiency gains that measure up to the secular pressures the system faces. So long as managed care relies on shell strategies to mete out one or another form of rationing, the only gains I see occurring are in medical mills, and in patient and physician frustration.

4. *While managed care is industrializing medical organization, science and technology are post-industrializing medical knowledge.* As medicine evolves, medical organization devolves. These conflicting trajectories reflect different principles of production. For medicine, value is produced by extending clinical capabilities. For managed care right now, value is produced by rationing them. The key to the industrial dynamics currently driving managed care is not the growth of bureaucracy. It is the division established between the technical and decision-making spheres of the physician role. The emphasis on discounts, on preauthorization, on gatekeepers doing at least some of the work of specialists, on utilization management, and on withholds and risk pools incentivizing clinical behavior, are all designed to control physician decision making so rationing in the technical sphere supports cost containment. Under these circumstances, managed care may well reduce the aggregate volume of physician—particularly specialty—services. It will not, however, elevate the productive capacity of the physician role. The problem is not with managed care, though. It is with the industrial logic managed care brings to *medical organization.* Since rationing is inconsistent with the principles of production that motivate *medicine,* it should not exist in medical organization. Therefore, I don't believe "industry" conditions in healthcare will significantly improve until managed care is post-industrialized, extending physicians' productive capacity through science and technology rather than limiting it through rationing.

Element # 2: Post-Industrialize the Doctor-Patient Relationship

Despite the changes managed care has brought to medicine, the doctor-patient relationship remains at the center of healthcare delivery. To use Ohmae's term, it is the key objective function in the industry—where the ultimate purpose of medicine resides, and where most health expenditures are generated. Yet, business strategy in managed care has neglected this all-important aspect of medicine. Even though some HMOs and PPOs have begun to formally address such related issues as clinical outcomes and patient satisfaction, the role of the doctor-patient relationship has received little, if any, strategic attention. Currently, for example, as was the case 10, 50, and a 100 years ago, the patient visits the doctor, the doctor diagnoses and treats, and the patient leaves the doctor. The only thing that has changed, really, is the complexity of organization and intensity of service inside the doctor-patient frame. Strategic thinking has not rethought the doctor-patient frame itself, *nor reworked how that frame fits in the value chains of different systems of managed care.*

I would attribute this to three intellectual tendencies in the current healthcare environment: 1) tacit acceptance of the classic professional model defining the physician role; 2) being either unprepared or unwilling to come up with different ways for meeting the requirements of detachment, trust, and transference in the doctor-patient relationship; and 3) a bias to impose controls on physicians in their existing professional role, rather than reengineer how the total system operates. If you think of the physician role as the engine of healthcare delivery, managed care is "flooring" the gas peddle of an engine built at the beginning of the century. Arguably, one of the most important lessons managed care can draw from a post-industrial economy is that the engine should be modernized. *Informationalizaton* is at the center of modernization of the physician role.

From primitive society to the present, the physician role has always revolved around the application of expert knowledge to patient care. At crucial points, however, the structural relationship between expert knowledge and the physician role has changed. In primitive society, the witch doctor interpreted supernatural processes the gods controlled. In effect, the witch doctor functioned as a *translator*. Starting with the Hippocratic tradition in ancient Greece and continuing to the present, doctors interpreted natural processes they presumed to control. These conditions defined the physician as a *technician*. Now that the tools of a post-industrial economy surround medicine, computer power drives the storage, retrieval, and interpretation of medical information physicians can then apply. Thus, the physician role has been recast into an *information manager*. While the evolution from translator to technician to information manager does not mean the first two roles are obsolete, it does suggest the first two roles should be subsumed under the role of information manager.

Davis makes the point that the economic value of information content in goods and services is growing faster than the economic value of goods and services themselves. His message is that smart versions of products and services have a competitive advantage over not-so-smart versions. I would extend this to the doctor-patient relationship. *Those managed care systems that use the physician role to create and sustain a smart version of the doctor-patient relationship should have a competitive advantage over those that don't.*

What's the difference between smart and not-so-smart doctor-patient relationships? The answer has much less to do with the quantity of information than with the extent to which information is leveraged. The standard doctor-patient relationship is episodic in nature. It is not so smart because information isn't leveraged. Patients go to the doctor when a problem has gotten to a certain level of intolerance, and the information generated, including outside tests and consults, is fixed in time and space. Expert elements of the information flow produce value, but only as a function of the intrinsic link between episodic patient care and fee-for-service. Notwithstanding a physician's clinical skills, *medicine's* productive capacity is limited to the absolute number of patient visits a physician can accommodate. The persistence of rationing in managed care attests to the inherent deficiencies of this model.

A smart relationship, on the other hand, leverages expert information before, during, and after the episodic doctor-patient encounter. Rather than being fixed in time and space, it operates on an "any time" production standard, making expert information available to patients in as close to real time as possible. In Chapter 5, I attributed the doctor-patient relationship to the *operations* value activity—the second of five value activities in the generic business system Porter describes. *What Davis' argument suggests is that in a post-industrial economy, the technological means exist for the doctor-patient relationship to be reconfigured so expert knowledge traditionally confined to a fixed frame of time and space can work any time.* When expert knowledge works any time, information is leveraged throughout the value chain, and the doctor-patient relationship becomes smart. In that sense, the distinction between smart and not-so-smart doctor-patient relationships reflects a distinction between healthcare delivery operating according to post-industrial versus industrial principles.

Drawing on Marilyn Ferguson, Davis suggests that the hologram is a metaphor for describing the organization of information flow in the post-industrial context. "For our purposes, the hologram has a very unique property. If the image is broken, any part of it will reconstruct the whole." This is important, Davis suggests, because, quoting Ferguson, it means "the whole code exists at every point in the medium" (1987, 142). Davis relates the hologram model of information flow to a *mass customizing* trend in post-industrial production. "CAD/CAM, for example, makes possible instantaneous changes in . . . specifications (and) customized adjustments . . . without any machine downtime. The general message is the more a company can deliver customized goods on a mass basis relative to the competition, the greater the competitive advantage" (1987, 157).

Turning now to the doctor-patient relationship, I would argue that the smart version—the post-industrial version—leverages the physician's role as information manager so the information elements of diagnosis, treatment, and follow-up can themselves be mass-customized and available to patients any time. The practical requirement is an unbundling and seamless re-integration of the physician role across the managed care value chain so patients receive both individual and standardized expert input at any point in the process. Figure 6–3 presents my depiction of a holographic information pathway associated with the doctor-patient relationship under a post-industrial managed care value chain. This contrasts with the linear information pathway of the industrial managed care value chain shown earlier in Chapter 5.

Element # 3: Post-Industrialize the Managed Care Value Chain

Post-industrializing the doctor-patient relationship involves reconfiguring the physician role to more fully leverage expert information. Post-industrializing the managed care value chain involves reconfiguring larger organizational frameworks to make medicine more productive. The two developments go hand in hand.

Davis and Davidson distinguish between *intra*organizations and *inter*organizations and suggest that in a post-industrial economy the movement should be towards the latter. The potential for interorganizations is tied to information technology that allows organizations to become electronically linked— backward to suppliers and forward, through distributors, to customers (1991, 132). Jim Manzi, Chairman and CEO of Lotus Development Cor-

Figure 6–3.   Post-Industrial versus Industrial Managed Care Value Chains

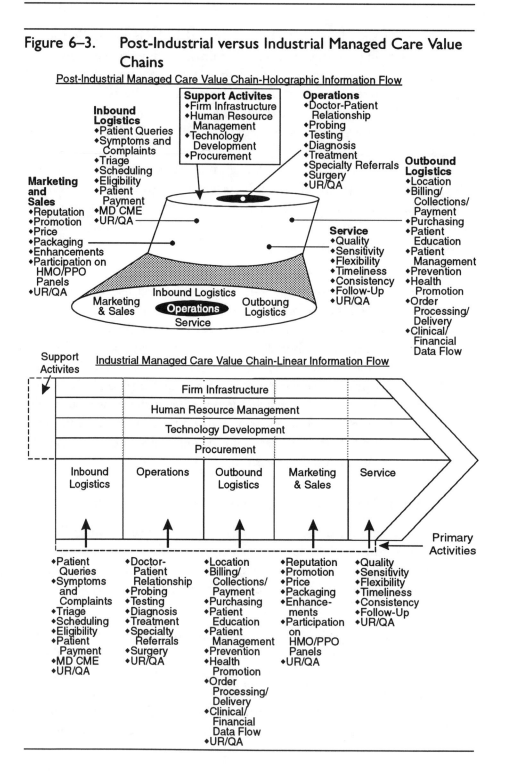

Post-Industrial Managed Care Value Chain-Holographic Information Flow

Support Activites
♦Firm Infrastructure
♦Human Resource Management
♦Technology Development
♦Procurement

Operations
♦Doctor-Patient Relationship
♦Probing
♦Testing
♦Diagnosis
♦Treatment
♦Specialty Referrals
♦Surgery
♦UR/QA

Inbound Logistics
♦Patient Queries
♦Symptoms and Complaints
♦Triage
♦Scheduling
♦Eligibility
♦Patient Payment
♦MD CME
♦UR/QA

Marketing and Sales
♦Reputation
♦Promotion
♦Price
♦Packaging
♦Enhancements
♦Participation on HMO/PPO Panels
♦UR/QA

Outbound Logistics
♦Location
♦Billing/ Collections/ Payment
♦Purchasing
♦Patient Education
♦Patient Management
♦Prevention
♦Health Promotion
♦Order Processing/ Delivery
♦Clinical/ Financial Data Flow

Service
♦Quality
♦Sensitivity
♦Flexibility
♦Timeliness
♦Consistency
♦Follow-Up
♦UR/QA

Marketing & Sales   Operations   Outbound Logistics
Inbound Logistics   Service

Industrial Managed Care Value Chain-Linear Information Flow

Support Activites

Firm Infrastructure
Human Resource Management
Technology Development
Procurement

| Inbound Logistics | Operations | Outbound Logistics | Marketing & Sales | Service |

Primary Activities

♦Patient Queries
♦Symptoms and Complaints
♦Triage
♦Scheduling
♦Eligibility
♦Patient Payment
♦MD CME
♦UR/QA

♦Doctor-Patient Relationship
♦Probing
♦Testing
♦Diagnosis
♦Treatment
♦Specialty Referrals
♦Surgery
♦UR/QA

♦Location
♦Billing/ Collections/ Payment
♦Purchasing
♦Patient Education
♦Patient Management
♦Prevention
♦Health Promotion
♦Order Processing/ Delivery
♦Clinical/ Financial Data Flow
♦UR/QA

♦Reputation
♦Promotion
♦Price
♦Packaging
♦Enhancements
♦Participation on HMO/PPO Panels
♦UR/QA

♦Quality
♦Sensitivity
♦Flexibility
♦Timeliness
♦Consistency
♦Follow-Up
♦UR/QA

poration addresses this same point when he refers to the "electronic keiretsu." In Japan, *keiretsu* means linkage. Post-war Japanese success has long been attributed, at least in part, to the *keiretsu* system of interlocking directorates comprised of the economy's leading manufacturers, banks, scientific establishments, and political leaders. In the United States, Manzi suggests, the electronic keiretsu represents a new way for companies to form information age interlocking directorates, allowing them to collaborate, pool resources, and coordinate more efficiently.[10]

The interorganizational model Davis and Davidson refer to and the electronic keiretsu Manzi refers to both speak to the vision of a post-industrial managed care value chain. Clearly, hospitals, physicians, ancillary suppliers, HMOs, PPOs, TPAs, and other vendors in UR, medical billing, and database management do not suffer from a shortage of computer power. But at the same time, computer power has not enabled managed care to advance the productive capacity of medicine. As *Consumer Reports* put it in a special series of articles on healthcare in the United States: "Of the 24 industrialized countries making up the Organization for Economic Cooperation and Economic Development (OECD), the U.S. spends more than twice as much on health per capita as the average. And it devotes a far greater percentage of its gross national product to healthcare than any other country. Yet, the other OECD countries—with the exception of Turkey and Greece, by far the poorest of the group—all have roughly as many doctors and hospitals per capita as we do. As for health status, of the 24 OECD countries, the U.S. ranks: 21st in infant mortality; 17th in male life expectancy; and 16th in female life expectancy." Drawing on the research of Dr. Barbara Starfield of Johns Hopkins who compared the United States with nine industrialized European nations around such indicators as quality primary care, infant mortality/life expectancy, and overall public satisfaction with the value of healthcare, *Consumer Reports* concluded that, "In all three areas, the U.S. ranked at or near the bottom."[11]

The message here is that it is one thing for electronic technology to operate in managed care. It is quite another to increase medicine's productivity. I

---

[10]Jim Manzi. "Computer Keiretsu: Japanese Idea, U.S. Style." *New York Times* (February 6, 1994): Section 3/Business, 15.

[11]*Consumer Reports* (July 1992): 445, 447; also see Paul Spector. "Failure, By the Numbers." *New York Times* (September 24, 1994): 19.

believe the more electronic technology operates within *intra*organizational managed care frameworks, the more fiefdoms, turf issues, and bureaucratic controls will limit medicine's productivity—further casting the spell of Malthus over medicine. Conversely, the more electronic technology operates in *inter*organizational managed care frameworks, the more medicine's productivity can increase. Perhaps *the* essential element making managed care interorganizational and medicine more productive is a restructuring of the space between provider/ producers and patient/consumers.

Turning back to the first part of this chapter, Davis develops three points about producer/consumer relationships in post-industrial economies that relate directly to the managed care value chain:

❑ First, the power of electronic technology coupled with the trend towards miniaturization allows production in a growing number of economic spheres to move further and further into the physical space of consumers.

❑ Second, consumers are more likely to purchase products they can have with them wherever they are, rather than purchase competing products they have to go to, to use. The more they can have products "any time, any where" the more effective those products will be for the end user.[12]

❑ Third, as the evolution from craft to industrial production required an expanded division of labor, evolution from industrial to post-industrial production requires an informationalized division of labor. Where intermediation increased efficiency under industrial conditions, it creates inefficiency under post-industrial conditions. *Informationalization plus disintermediation*, therefore, should be strategic objectives under post-industrial production.

For managed care, this suggests that *smart business strategy ought to focus on pushing operations—physicians and other providers—down the value chain to bring medical knowledge as close to the patient as possible.* In addition, the

---

[12]The "any time, any where" standard is prominent in the telecommunications industry right now and relates directly to AT&T's acquisition of McCaw Cellular Communications. A *Wall Street Journal* article referred to this aspect of AT&T's strategy explicitly: McCaw "might help American Telephone & Telegraph Co.'s 'any where, any time' communications strategy . . . " See John Keller. "AT&T Wants McCaw to Be Omnipresent." *The Wall Street Journal* (August 27, 1993): B1.

value chain needs to be informationalized so the physician role manages expert knowledge according to an any time production standard. The more medicine functions as an input throughout the value chain, the more productive it becomes. Certainly, these are speculative themes. Nevertheless, if the organizational side of American medicine is to do justice to its clinical capabilities, in my judgment these themes have to become part of the conventional logic of strategic thinking in managed care. The following three examples illustrate ways in which the value chain could be post-industrialized:

1. **Informationalize the House Call.** It used to be that the doctor's black bag symbolized the house call, but as times changed home visits simply became too inefficient. With patients having a monitor and modem at home, though, doctors can make their house call without ever leaving the office. Harvard Community Health Plan is experimenting with just such a program. "The plan has placed terminals in homes of 150 members in an experiment to both promote health education and reduce unnecessary doctor visits. More than 30 percent of appointments are made for maladies that would cure themselves without doctor intervention," according to the associate medical director of the HMO. "When patients dial up the data base and type in symptoms, they get a series of questions that lead either to recommendations for home treatment or to make an appointment. If a member's answers indicate the possibility of serious illness, an alarm sounds at the clinic, alerting staff members to call the home."[13] The informationalized house call allows patients to have real-time access to expert information without an office visit. While this is not necessary for everyone, for parents with young children, those with chronic illnesses, and the elderly—particularly young elders (age 55 to 75)—the informationalized house call has the capacity to make medicine a lot more productive.

2. **Informationalize the Physician Role.** The informationalized house call is just one example of post-industrializing the managed care value chain. A second and related example, following the

13Ron Winslow. "Desktop Doctors." *The Wall Street Journal* (April 6, 1992): R14.

holographic metaphor discussed above, involves literally informationalizing how a physician conducts clinical business. Informationalizing, in this sense goes beyond automating medical records to automating as much of the elemental activities feeding into and flowing out of the doctor-patient encounter as possible. A medical director of an HMO I speak with on occasion refers to such a system as the "black box." The "black box" should be capable of automating what doctors have traditionally retained in their heads, committed to paper flow, and delegated to office staff. "Black box" functions include, but would not be limited to, 1) screens for history taking and diagnosis; 2) protocols and decision trees delimiting the appropriate course of action; 3) entries for lab tests, medications, ancillary support, and patient progress; and 4) medical record coordination, transfer, and retrieval between a patient's primary care doctor and specialists. More than just logging information, which is beginning to occur in certain select hospitals with the PC at the patient's bedside, the "black box" should be capable of thinking, tracking, and assigning information—not to supplant physicians, but to make them more productive.[14]

3. **Informationalize Principles of Production in Managed Care.**
   The prevailing view is that the power of information systems is their capacity to attack healthcare inflation: First, by tracking utilization, profiling providers, and identifying where overutilization is occurring; second, by reducing the paper bureaucracy in claims processing; and third, by informing payors (carriers and employers) about procedure costs, where their money is going, and what outcomes eventually occurred. My own view is that these gains are secondary to the transformation in production capabilities that automated information systems represents for managed care. Currently, classic bureaucratic principles of organization are at the center of production in all managed care systems—bureaucratic organization is what makes a doctor's office, hospital, and HMO or PPO tick. Automate *that* production process by informationalizing the linkages between and within value activities in the value

---

[14]See Winslow. "Desktop Doctors." and Glen Rifkin. "New Momentum for Electronic Patient Records." *New York Times* (May 2, 1993): F8.

chain and production will occur at an entirely different level. Transformation of this sort is analogous to progressing from the horse and buggy to the automobile. The automobile here, though, is not just the information superhighway, it is an intelligent system with the capacity to *produce* far in excess of the standard managed care bureaucracies.

While these systems are still developing, as an article in the *The Wall Street Journal* put it, "The era of intelligent computer networks . . . is officially underway." The article refers to "Telecript," a product developed by a consortium including AT&T and General Magic, that "allows computer users to easily send electronic agents out on computer networks to find and filter information" and to send agents "far away to operate on your behalf."[15] If adapted for healthcare delivery, it suggests the potential for the managed care value chain to function as an *automated, integrated system*. Such a system should have an information pathway with functions that log, track, combine, and evaluate clinical data, plus recommend a course of action—all still under the supervision and control of physicians. Already, computer programs exist that "link healthcare providers such as physicians, hospitals and pharmacies with managed care organizations and health plan sponsors." At the push of a button, these programs allow physicians to compare the cost of alternative therapies, check to see if a prescription has been filled, retrieve lab results and images from X-rays or electrocardiograms, and update as well as review the patient's medical record.[16]

Recasting the principles of production in managed care along these lines makes medicine more productive in three key ways: 1) it gives physicians more direct patient contact with cases where their clinical judgment, skills, and experience are most needed; 2) it allows more patient data on more

---

[15]Christian Hill. "New Software Helps Networks Get Smarter." *The Wall Street Journal* (January 6, 1994): B1; also see Christian Hill. "Electronic 'Agents' Bring Virtual Shopping A Bit Closer to Reality." *The Wall Street Journal* (September 27, 1994): A1.

[16]See "McKesson's PCS Unit Agrees to Buy a Stake in Integrated Medical." *The Wall Street Journal* (January 18, 1994): B4; and Ron Winslow. "Computers Helping Doctors Match Care With Costs Can Lower Bills, Study Says." *The Wall Street Journal* (January 20, 1993): B6.

patients to be collected, organized, and reviewed by nurses, technical support staff, and physicians in a timely and efficient manner; and 3) it enables expert knowledge for diagnosis and treatment as well as managing chronic illness to be available to patients any time.

Element # 4: Post-Industrialize Organization in Managed Care

The old saying, "The more things change, the more they remain the same," doesn't necessarily apply to organization in post-industrial economies. No doubt, there are many ways in which the industrial/post-industrial divide has not changed the nature and character of organization. Budgets, leadership, accountability, responsibility, span of control, administration, and politics all somehow remain a constant. And there are other constants as well. But since the scientific and technological possibilities have changed, the functions that organization is supposed to address have also changed. These changes frame the fourth and last element to be discussed in this outline of post-industrial strategic thinking for managed care.

In distinguishing "business" from "organization," Davis and Davidson make a point that senior executives may not want to hear. They ask, "Do you and your company spend less than two-thirds of your time and energies on your business, and more than one-third on your organization?" If so, they argue, "then you have a business that exists to support an organization, not an organization that exists to support a business. It may be time to kill your organization before it kills your business" (1991, 112)[17] They relate this observation to Henderson's growth/share matrix described in Chapter 4, saying that just as there are "dogs" in business, there are "dogs" in organization. "Aging organizations are dogs, biting the business hand that feeds them, and should also be discarded" (1991, 119). However, while executives may be quick to say "My product line is aging—I need next generation products," they seem unable to say, "My organization is aging—I need the next generation organization" (1991, 121). Businesses are most likely to be successful if their organization is congruent with the life cycle of their business (1991, 122). Because this is usually not possible, though, *Businesses should stay just a little bit ahead of their organizations*" (1991, 125).

---

[17]Also see Davis, 197.

Staying just a little ahead of the organization may sound simple enough, but it's not all that common in healthcare. In my own community, for example, two local hospitals recently initiated major layoffs to cope with the discounts required by area HMOs and PPOs. These layoffs were part of an explicit "restructuring" intended to lower costs by phasing out LPNs in favor of a new nursing category: The PCA or patient care associate. The more lower-wage PCAs replace LPNs and lower-wage LPNs replace RNs, the more money the two hospitals expect to save. One hospital president, putting a positive spin on the layoffs, was quoted as saying, "To survive, you have got to be incredibly innovative in improving quality and cutting costs. . . . What we are committed to in this organization is to improve the value to the patient."[18] The two hospitals are certainly not alone in relying on lower-cost substitutes to reduce overhead. In fact, this approach is rapidly gaining acceptance in the industry.[19] But do these actions lead to a true "restructuring"? Are they "incredibly innovative"? Are they "improving value"? I would answer no on all counts because in each instance change is directed to the "organization" not the "business."

Take restructuring. It doesn't take a rocket scientist to know that revenues should exceed costs. While hospital layoffs may have brought each organization's costs back in line with revenues, how was the hospitals' *business* restructured? Clinical programs were not phased out and new ones added based on a different approach to the market. Physician practices were not acquired and integrated in order to redesign hospital operations. No managed care, market, or informationalization initiative was adopted to change the character and content of the hospitals' four walls. In short, neither hospital transformed its business. The focus was on hospital organization, with the organization being paired back to meet the diminishing revenues the existing business generated.

Compare the above response to two other healthcare industry situations where reducing costs was also considered crucial to continued success, but in each instance *changes in organization followed changes in the business.*

---

[18]Glenn Blain. "Hospitals Facing Cost-Cutting Pressures." *Rockland Journal News* (January 10, 1994): A1.

[19]See George Anders. "Nurses Decry Cost-Cutting Plan That Uses Aides to Do More Jobs." *The Wall Street Journal* (January 20, 1994): B1.

❑ In the first case, Columbia/HCA, now the world's largest investor-owned hospital group, has been pursuing an acquisition strategy targeting multiple, often troubled, hospitals by geographic market. Once acquired, restructuring involves integrating and consolidating operations, eliminating duplication, closing beds, investing in new clinical services, developing equity relationships with physicians, leveraging purchasing power with vendors, and linking much leaner hospital platforms with other medical services to deliver "one-stop shopping."[20] While Columbia is a national corporation, comparable strategies with somewhat different emphases are underway in specific cities. In St. Louis, for instance, a megamerger involving Barnes Hospital, Jewish Hospital, and Christian Hospital has enabled the parent corporation to selectively integrate services, reduce overhead, and develop a managed care delivery system capable of rivaling Blue Cross or any of the commercial or for-profit HMOs in town. And in Boston, five of the city's major teaching institutions, all affiliated with Harvard Medical School—Brigham and Women's Hospital, Massachusetts General, Children's, Beth Israel, and New England Deaconess—are pursuing various forms of collaboration to in some combination merge, consolidate, eliminate, and develop specialty services.[21] No doubt, all of these situations involve layoffs. But in each, changes in hospital organization are intended to follow changes in the hospital business.

❑ In the second case, Merck, a leading drugmaker, acquired Medco, an industry leader in mail-order pharmaceutical distribution. The acquisition enabled Merck to restructure its method of sales to powerful managed care networks.[22] As *The Wall Street Journal* reported, "Take a database detailing millions of drug prescriptions. Ask your computer which ones can be switched to your company's drugs. Employ pharmacists to suggest the switches to patients' doctors. That's the prescrip-

---

[20]See Milt Freudenheim. "Cashing In on Healthcare's Troubles." *New York Times* (July 21, 1991): F1; Katheryn Jones. "A Hospital Giant Comes to Town, Bringing Change." *New York Times* (November 21, 1993): F4; and Allen Meyerson. "Now It's the Rick Scott Health Plan." *New York Times* (October 30, 1994): 3:1.

[21]See David Stipp. "Five Hospitals Plan to Discuss Joining Services." *The Wall Street Journal* (July 1, 1993): B6.

[22]See George Anders. "Managed Healthcare Jeopardizes Outlook For Drug 'Detailers.'" *The Wall Street Journal* (September 10, 1993): A1.

tion for marketing success behind Merck & Co.'s . . . acquisition of Medco Containment Services, Merck officials say. And despite concern about patient privacy, this high tech strategy is expected to set the marketing pattern for the industry. When the Tiffany of drug makers agreed . . . to pay $6 billion for the Wal-Mart of pills, Merck was buying much more than a mail-order drug company. It was buying Medco's technology and information."[23] Six months after the merger, Merck took the unprecedented step of preparing to enter into "capitation and other risk-sharing arrangements" with HMOs.[24] Merck then, no less than others in the healthcare industry, experienced revenue losses and other setbacks due to the impact of managed care. But Merck changed its business before it changed its organization, and it didn't pass off organizational changes for changes in its business either.[25]

Post-industrializing managed care organization means changing business first and organization second. As the Merck-Medco case illustrates, however, it also means transforming business based on the productive capacities of the information age. Though the focus of most of this chapter, and indeed most of this book, has been on physicians and managed care systems, the follow-ing *post-industrial strategy check list* illustrates the kind of questions all health-

---

[23]Elyse Tanouye. "Merck Will Exploit Medco's Data Base." *The Wall Street Journal* (August, 4, 1993): B1.

[24]Elyse Tanouye. "Merck Officials Suggest Drug Maker Will Aim for Generic Market Overseas." *The Wall Street Journal* (February 14, 1994): B5.

[25]As a consequence of Merck's acquisition of Medco, other pharmaceutical giants have been forced to rework their businesses by, in most instances, acquiring drug benefit firms of their own and integrating them into their basic operation. Eli Lilly's acquisition of PCS Health Systems, SmithKline Beecham's acquisition of Diversified Pharmaceutical Services, and Pfizer's strategic alliance with Value Health's ValueRx are all examples of leading pharmaceutical players' attempts to restructure the conduct of their business. See, Ron Winslow and Stephen Moore. "SmithKline Sets to Purchase Benefits Firm." *The Wall Street Journal* (May 4, 1994): A3; Milt Freudenheim. "A Shift in Power in Pharmaceuticals." *New York Times* (May 9, 1994): D1; Milt Freudenheim. "Pharmaceutical Giant Is Buying Operator of Drug-Benefit Plans." *New York Times* (July 12, 1994): A1; Thomas Burton and Elyse Tanouye. "Eli Lilly to Buy McKesson Unit For $4 Billion." *The Wall Street Journal* (July 12, 1994): A3; Stephanie Mehta. "In Shadow of Medco and PCS, Other Firms Are Busy." *The Wall Street Journal* (July 13, 1994): B2; and Elyse Tanouye and Greg Steinmetz. "Managed Care Feeding Frenzy Probably Hasn't Ended." *The Wall Street Journal* (July 13, 1994): B3.

care industry players should be asking about their business and their organization in a post-industrial economy:

- ❑ What's core and what's peripheral to the business, and how can informationalization either refine or redefine the business?

- ❑ What tangible products and services can be made intangible, and in what ways can the integration of information content in such products and services increase their effectiveness and efficiency?

- ❑ How can the constraints of time, place, and space within organization be reduced by information technology?

- ❑ Where can informational linkages within and between value activities of the value chain and between the producer and consumer's value chain most significantly reduce intermediation in the production process?

- ❑ How can organization enable different value activities to produce more value in the same space or the same value in less space?

- ❑ How can production be brought closer to the consumer's space in distribution and sales to approximate an any time production standard?

- ❑ Where in both the business and the organization can informationalization and intangibility create a sustainable edge over one's tangible-oriented competitors?

POST-INDUSTRIALIZING MANAGED CARE: A REPRISE

One of the great ironies of modernity is that the more impressive science becomes, the less certainty there is about its purpose and direction. This dynamic is doubly ironic in medicine because medical science is so clearly grounded in improving the human condition. Davis takes a stab at part of this problem with his argument that organizations typically, and often persistently, lag behind scientific and technological capabilities. What Davis does not say, though, but is a point commentators have long noted, is that advances in science and technology change an organization's functional requirements; and the more significant the functional change in organizations, the more resistance is promulgated by existing stakeholders with something to lose. At least a partial explanation for the loss of meaning that follows in the wake of modernity, then, can be traced to the gulf between what is scientifically and technically possible and what actually exists, a gulf that in large measure results from good old-fashioned self-interest. For post-industrial strategic thinking to succeed in medicine, it will have to present the case for functional change in a way that redirects self-interest.

Two observations about self-interest under managed care deserve mention here. The first centers on action, the second on structure.

Action

Managed care has sparked considerable entrepreneurial activity in American medicine. In Porter's terms, this reflects a change from buyer to supplier domination in the medical marketplace. With the purchasing clout wielded by large managed care networks, hospitals and physicians no longer hold the upper hand. Whether because of DRG reimbursement, competitive policies in the Reagan years, or the lure of Wall Street, hospitals long ago responded to the growing bargaining power of buyers through mergers, acquisitions, alliances, and group purchasing arrangements. For physicians, though, the story is different. While a relatively small number invested in laboratories, imaging facilities, and freestanding surgery centers during the 1980s, it was Clinton's election in 1992 that pushed physicians as a class to become more entrepreneurial.

Since the Clinton endorsement of managed care, "contracting" in some form has become, arguably, *the* most widespread entrepreneurial activity among physicians. As discussed earlier, contracting refers to participating or par agreements between payors and providers. The original Blue Cross and Blue Shield model was based on individual Cross and Shield plans having par agreements with hospitals and physicians. Similarly, the Medicare program is based on par agreements. All managed care networks, in fact, are predicated on par agreements. Where HMOs and PPOs pursued contracting to build provider networks for enrolling members, physicians now pursue contracting to channel HMO/PPO members to a narrower band of practices. In its purest form, contracting involves managed care systems entering into exclusive agreements with either single-specialty provider networks, or multispecialty IPAs, PHOs, and medical groups.

The current trend is for contracting to be linked to MSOs that not only provide insurance industry functions such as claims processing, utilization review, and data reporting, but also support physicians' medical office functions. MSOs, then, operate in three contexts: 1) in IPAs, PHOs, medical groups, and single provider networks to address the administrative requirements of capitation and other managed care arrangements; 2) in hospitals to manage and/or purchase physicians' practices for referrals as well as to administer managed care contracts; and 3) in non-bricks-and-mortar medical group practices, often called "group practice without walls."

Groups without walls are initiated by physicians so they can remain in their private offices and realize most of the autonomy they enjoyed previously. But now they function as a profit center within a larger group. The MSO is the administrative core that ties together and supports each of the practices or profit centers of the group. The profit centers themselves result from physicians exchanging the value of their existing practice for stock in the newly formed group practice. Since the group is incorporated and organized to function as an economically integrated unit, its physicians are legally able to pursue two core objectives: Include additional services such as imaging centers, labs, and medical supply companies as revenue centers within the group; and package the group's entire product portfolio for contracting purposes in negotiations with HMOs and other managed care payors.[26]

What I would emphasize about all such entrepreneurial activity, however, is that *it does not and will not fundamentally change the underlying grammar of private practice, fee-for-service medicine, which the majority of American physicians, even those in small, medium, and many large groups, continue to embrace.* In fact, I would argue that most physicians' entrepreneurial activity represents nothing more than a readjustment of the traditional private practice environment to the realities of managed care.

In my judgment, the more physicians pursue their entrepreneurial interests without fundamentally changing their business objectives in the private practice environment, the more the dictates of cost containment in managed care will be imposed upon them. Given the propensities of episodic

---

[26]For descriptions and thougtful practical discussions bearing on the development and operation of MSOs see two volumes: Keith Korenchuk. *Transforming the Delivery of Healthcare: The Integration Process* (Englewood, CO: Medical Group Management Association, 1994); and Bette Waddington, editor. *Integration Issues in Physician/Hospital Affiliations* (Englewood, CO: Medical Group Management Association, 1993).

patient care and fee-for-service medicine, if physicians and managed care systems are ever to move beyond the divergent interests of their respective spheres, it will have to be through a rethinking of function and functional relationships on both sides. The key to that rethinking, I believe, is more likely to be found in new kinds of partnerships, productivity objectives, and synergies articulated through post-industrial strategic thinking, than anywhere else.

Structure

Aside from the different actions that physicians and managed care systems engage in—the former trying to earn more; the latter, trying to pay less—there is an important structural distinction as well. Physicians as actors pursue interests from the bottom up. HMOs and PPOs as institutions impose interests from the top down. No matter how you look at it, physicians operate in institutional frameworks that HMOs, PPOs, and other managed care systems establish. If those frameworks are deficient, it sets into motion actions and reactions that shape overall performance.

Based on my remarks in Chapter 5, I believe a serious deficiency exists in the HMO sector. While HMOs are supposed to pay for *and* deliver medical services, most in fact just pay for services and contract with physicians who deliver them. Since those physicians conduct themselves according to private practice, fee-for-service principles of organization, the productive capabilities HMOs presuppose have not been realized. As competitive pressures force HMOs to bear down on provider panels to control costs, they invariably chip away at physicians' income and time-honored independence. Inevitably, the system's inflationary spiral is mirrored in a separate spiral of physician resentment.

Turning back to the Porter discussion in Chapter 5, I'm convinced that the nub of the problem involves how *production* under managed care *is organized*. Recall that for Porter, production centers on the *operations value activity* and operations involves "(a)ctivities associated with transforming inputs into their final product form, such as machining, packaging, assembly, equipment maintenance, testing, printing and facility operations."[27] In healthcare,

---

[27]Michael E. Porter. *Competitive Advantage: Creating and Sustaining Superior Performance* (New York: The Free Press, 1985), 40.

no aspect of the system is more important for transforming inputs into their final product form than the doctor-patient relationship. The physician treating patients *is* the operations value activity that drives the industry. But, and this is a big but, since all PPOs and at least 9 out of 10 HMOs are organized around participating providers in private practice, almost all of managed care is prevented from exercising direct control over *the production process* the entire industry depends on.

From the standpoint of managed care generally, there are four structural implications I would emphasize:

1. PPOs, POS plans, and most HMOs are fundamentally the same when it comes to production: They all depend on physician networks to deliver health services. How these managed care systems use their value chains to produce different kinds of superior value, not how their benefit designs vary, should be the primary basis for differentiation in the marketplace.

2. All managed care systems—with the exception of staff and salaried group model HMOs—should avoid concentrating on the operations value activity in their value chain and should concentrate instead on inbound logistics, outbound logistics, marketing and sales, or service. That is, they should concentrate on those value activities they can best fashion to produce superior value.

3. Staff and salaried group model HMOs should concentrate first and foremost on the operations value activity. To the extent that absolute superiority is not achieved in the operations value activity, these HMOs neglect their historic role under managed care.

4. All network-based HMOs that concentrate on the operations value activity will only alienate the providers they depend on. This alienation can be traced to informationalized bureaucracies that impose utilization management procedures on physicians that such HMOs do not and cannot directly control.

From the standpoint of post-industrial strategy, three additional structural implications should be emphasized:

1. Compared to PPOs, industry logic dictates that HMOs have a firmer grip on their provider networks, are more committed to using infrastructure to achieve cost containment, and are more

inclined to extend their organization into the physician's office and members' everyday lives. Consequently, network-based HMOs should concentrate on value activities that *lessen the space between physician and patient.*

2. Since the business of network-based HMOs requires that they manage healthcare delivery indirectly, physicians are responsible to the HMO for services patients receive. The business of PPOs, on the other hand, is to simply establish discount arrangements through which members may purchase services. Under these circumstances, physicians are responsible not to the PPO but to the patient. Unlike HMOs, therefore, PPO value activities are much less involved in the actual processes of healthcare delivery, and should concentrate instead on *reducing the space between patient and payment.*

3. The standard that should be used to judge whether industry behavior under managed care supports the public interest is *whether systems of managed care make medicine productive in a manner that is commensurate with progress in the state of the art.* At the delivery system level, production depends on the different ways managed care systems organize their respective value chains. Within these value chains, production depends on different ways informationalization drives specific value activities. And in the marketplace, production depends on the information content of different tangible and intangible health services and how effective those services are in people's lives.

The three scenarios below illustrate how PPO and HMO value chains could be organized under post-industrial strategic thinking. A few caveats though: a) the scenarios are examples, not absolutes; b) many of the examples are themselves in the developing stage as of this writing; c) the overriding rationale for informationalization is not to capture data *ad nauseam*, but to drive value activities in order to make medicine more productive; d) similarities between Scenarios 1 and 2 result from PPOs and HMOs being network-based, while similarities between Scenarios 2 and 3 result from HMOs being capitated systems; and e) post-industrializing a value chain should be sequenced, with the goal being to establish functional competence, and then extend that competence to build a long-term competitive advantage. Decisions regarding functional objectives, priorities, and timing should all be shaped by the overall strategy.[28]

Scenario #1: PPO Value Chain

☐ **Inbound Logistics:** 1) require credit card use and electronic claims processing with preferred providers, and credit card use when possible with nonpreferred providers; 2) establish holistic provider panels (e.g., chiropractors, nutritionists, and acupuncturists; and 3) package discount fee and benefit arrangements for selected vertical services (e.g., pulmonary/allergy; orthopedic/chiropractic/physical therapy; and dentistry/vision/pharmacy/mental health); 4) maintain an on-line referral bureau for members to access information on providers; and 5) offer members the option of having the PPO negotiate arrangements with non-PPO specialists to reduce out-of-pocket costs.

☐ **Operations:** 1) monitor patient outcomes; 2) evaluate preferred provider quality of care; and 3) administer nonintrusive utilization review.

☐ **Outbound Logistics:** 1) mail comprehensive monthly statements showing charged and covered expenses, plus balance; 2) include periodic reminders about preventive services and savings opportunities in monthly statements; and 3) distribute customized health information reflecting members' utilization and risk profile.

☐ **Marketing and Sales:** 1) link PPO health insurance to other financial products such as life, disability, and long-term care insurance, mutual funds, and annuities by tying multiyear health expenditure savings to credits for other products; and 2) offer PPO members unique access to wellness, prevention, fitness, stress reduction, and other special services through their credit card.

---

[28]The scenarios do not address POS plans or out-of-panel HMOs because these are midrange products falling somewhere between PPOs and HMOs. Since the entire managed care continuum is undergoing continuous evolution, the illustrations for network-based HMOs and PPOs could be adopted and modified by these and other managed care systems.

❑ **Service:** 1) maintain a billing support function to develop payment plans for expensive out-of-panel and noncovered services; and 2) evaluate all member/PPO encounters.

Scenario #2: Network-Based HMO Value Chain

❑ **Inbound Logistics:** 1) maintain on-line, real-time capabilities for HMO members to ask questions concerning symptoms and schedule provider visits; 2) automate the triage function to scale back the PCP gatekeeper role and electronically refer patients to specialists or subspecialists for office visits; and 3) maintain and regularly update an integrated system of clinical protocols for physician use.

❑ **Operations:** 1) establish and maintain an automated medical record system linking PCPs, specialists, and subspecialists; 2) electronically transmit the updated record so it accompanies patients at any HMO physician encounter; 3) always send the updated record back to the member's PCP for review and storage; and 4) provide systems capabilities to increase physician office productivity and clinical effectiveness.

❑ **Outbound Logistics:** 1) establish electronic linkages between physician offices, hospitals, labs, pharmacies, and other ancillary providers to streamline data flow and clinical directives; 2) maintain an E-mail system between physician and patient for physicians to monitor patient compliance and track results; 3) maintain centralized systems to monitor patient outcomes, evaluate quality of care, and administer nonintrusive utilization review; and 4) profile physician performance and eliminate those who do not practice quality/cost-effective medicine.

❑ **Marketing and Sales:** 1) compile a comprehensive database on HMO members and segment membership by risk factors; 2) offer ongoing health promotion and prevention programs through holistic and allopathic initiatives; and 3) produce interactive cable programming to address specific chronic, stress, and lifestyle related issues.

❑ **Service:** 1) provide members with a healthcare credit card and include reminders about preventive services and savings opportunities in monthly statements; 2) maintain automated systems to ensure appropriate physician as well as patient follow-up; and 3) evaluate all member/HMO encounters.

Scenario #3: Staff and Salaried Group-Model HMO Value Chain

- ❑ **Inbound Logistics:** 1) organize PCPs, nurse practitioners, and physicians assistants into primary care teams; 2) maintain on-line, real-time system capabilities for member Q&As; 3) establish an automated office scheduling system; and 4) maintain an automated medical record system linking primary care teams, specialists, and subspecialists.

- ❑ **Operations:** 1) organize physician and ancillary staff by specialty (e.g., orthopedic, urology, cardiology) *and* product line (e.g., hypertension, asthma, headaches, lower back pain) production functions; 2) fully leverage specialty and subspecialty expertise; 3) incorporate alternative or nonallopathic providers in clinical division of labor; 4) standardize patient pathways and maintain automated data entry and patient tracking systems; 5) integrate the use of automated clinical protocols in all patient encounters; 6) establish formal mechanisms for rapid adoption of clinical, pharmacological, and biotechnology developments in day-to-day medical practice; and 7) use value engineering and value analysis techniques to evaluate all clinical performance.

- ❑ **Outbound Logistics:** 1) establish separate health promotion initiatives for chronic conditions; 2) maintain an E-mail system to monitor patient progress from medical visits and wellness programs; 3) maintain electronic linkages between physicians' offices, hospitals, labs, pharmacies, and other ancillary providers to streamline data flow and clinical directives; and 4) maintain centralized systems to evaluate quality of care and administer formal and systematic utilization review.

- ❑ **Marketing and Sales:** 1) compile a comprehensive database on HMO members and segment membership by risk factors; 2) offer ongoing health promotion and prevention programs through holistic and allopathic initiatives; and 3) produce interactive cable programming to address specific chronic, stress, and lifestyle related issues.

- ❑ **Service:** 1) provide members with a healthcare credit card and include reminders about preventive services and savings opportunities in monthly statements; 2) maintain order entry systems between members' homes, pharmacy, health stores, and other health service venues; 3) maintain automated systems to ensure appropriate physician and patient follow-up; and 4) evaluate all member/HMO encounters.

A FINAL NOTE

The mark of modern medicine is its extraordinary capacity to treat what once was the province of the gods. Insofar as rising costs associated with that capacity have themselves become an almost insurmountable burden to our economy, the problem is not with medicine per se, but with the way the business of medicine is organized. Viewed historically, medicine has always been a peculiar enterprise—a business, but also an institution in the public trust. Indeed, the tension between these two competing poles frame just about every chapter in the history of American medicine.

What is significant about the current chapter, is that at a time when medicine's potential is so great, the gulf between its ability to be productive and the organization of medical production has widened. The more high-tech medicine becomes, the more inflation sets in; whereas, the more high-tech other industries become, the more efficiency and savings set in.

While the present emphasis in both health policy and health insurance is on managed care and having systems of managed care compete with one another, no policy or industry reform will be effective until business strategy succeeds in making managed care systems produce better medical services at a lower cost *and* raises the health status of the covered population. For healthcare delivery to progress to that point, industry structure under managed care will have to evolve beyond the private practice, fee-for-service environment and its almost pre-economic links to piece-rate production. Business strategy, in other words, will have to push medicine towards a more ambitious production standard. Ironically, at a time when the reach of medical science is so great, it may well be the imagination and standards of business strategy in medicine that determines just what promise medical science holds for the future of American society.

APPENDIX A

The Strategic Thinking Model

Regardless of whether one's goal is to develop a strategic, market, or business plan, those who plan the best will be those with the best strategy. And the best strategy occurs when *strategic thinking* is relatively autonomous from the nuts and bolts of the actual planning process itself.

The analogy to architecture and construction is useful here. While an architect's thinking should clearly take into consideration the practical aspects and planning issues involved in construction, what sets the architect's thinking apart is concept and design, form and function. These then get formalized and implemented in the builder's actual workplans. Architects whose thinking is idealistic and removed from the end user's needs, not to mention the builder's costs, are not usually successful. Conversely, those whose creative distance allows them to formulate something special, as well as something that "works," are the most successful.

Each of the authors discussed above are superb architects—superb strategic thinkers. Figure A–1 takes a step back from their work and outlines a generic model for strategic thinking that all of the authors fit into. This model supports the development of strategy in strategic planning no less than market or business planning.[1]

---

1 The concept of a "strategic thinking model" is borrowed from James Webber and Joseph Peters. *Strategic Thinking: New Frontier for Hospital Management* (Chicago: American Hospital Association, 1983), 11.

Figure A–1. Strategic Thinking Model

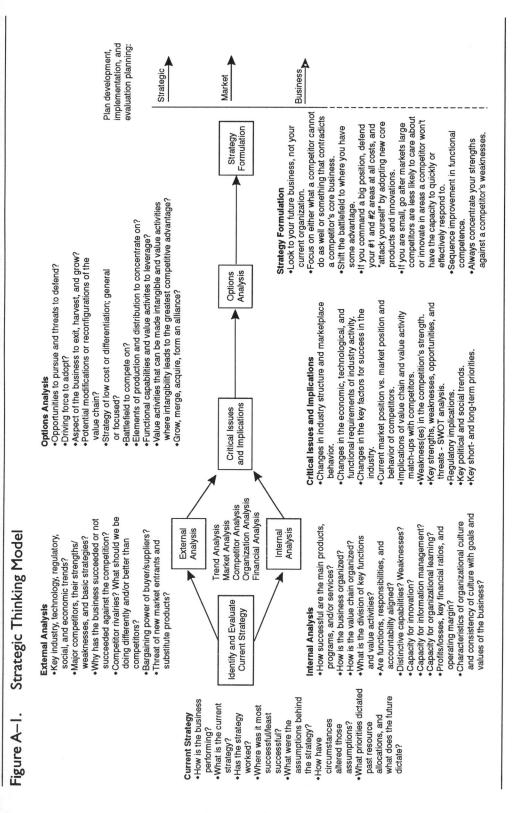

Plan development, implementation, and evaluation planning:

Strategic →

Market →

Business →

External Analysis
- Key industry, technology, regulatory, social, and economic trends?
- Major competitors, their strengths/weaknesses, and basic strategies?
- Why has the business succeeded or not succeeded against the competition?
- Competitor rivalries? What should we be doing differently and/or better than competitors?
- Bargaining power of buyer/suppliers?
- Threat of new market entrants and substitute products?

Options Analysis
- Opportunities to pursue and threats to defend?
- Driving force to adopt?
- Aspect of the business to exit, harvest, and grow?
- Potential modifications or reconfigurations of the value chain?
- Strategy of low cost or differentiation; general or focused?
- Battlefield to compete on?
- Elements of production and distribution to concentrate on?
- Functional capabilities and value activities to leverage?
- Value activities that can be made intangible and value activities where intangibility leads to the greatest competitive advantage?
- Grow, merge, acquire, form an alliance?

Strategy Formulation
- Look to your future business, not your current organization.
- Focus on either what a competitor cannot do as well or something that contradicts a competitor's core business.
- Shift the battlefield to where you have some advantage.
- If you command a big position, defend your #1 and #2 areas at all costs, and "attack yourself" by adopting new core products and innovations.
- If you are small, go after markets large competitors are less likely to care about or innovate in areas a competitor won't have the capacity to quickly or effectively respond to.
- Sequence improvement in functional competence.
- Always concentrate your strengths against a competitor's weaknesses.

Critical Issues and Implications
- Changes in industry structure and marketplace behavior.
- Changes in the economic, technological, and functional requirements of industry activity.
- Changes in the key factors for success in the industry.
- Current market position vs. market position and behavior of competitors.
- Implications of value chain and value activity match-ups with competitors.
- Weakness(es) in the competition's strength.
- Key strengths, weaknesses, opportunities, and threats - SWOT analysis.
- Regulatory implications.
- Key political and social trends.
- Key short- and long-term priorities.

Current Strategy
- How is the business performing?
- What is the current strategy?
- Has the strategy worked?
- Where was it most successful/least successful?
- What were the assumptions behind the strategy?
- How have circumstances altered those assumptions?
- What priorities dictated past resource allocations, and what does the future dictate?

External Analysis

Trend Analysis
Market Analysis
Competitor Analysis
Organization Analysis
Financial Analysis

Internal Analysis

Identify and Evaluate Current Strategy

Critical Issues and Implications

Options Analysis

Strategy Formulation

Internal Analysis
- How successful are the main products, programs, and/or services?
- How is the business organized?
- How is the value chain organized?
- What is the division of key functions and value activities?
- Are functions, responsibilities, and accountability aligned?
- Distinctive capabilities? Weaknesses?
- Capacity for innovation?
- Capacity for information management?
- Capacity for organizational learning?
- Profits/losses, key financial ratios, and operating margin?
- Characteristics of organizational culture and consistency of culture with goals and values of the business?

APPENDIX B

Industry Matrices and Strategy

The product portfolio matrices originated by The Boston Consulting Group and reviewed in Chapter 4 represent one technique that can help inform strategy development. A second technique focuses on a company's market position and industry attractiveness. Porter attributes this technique to General Electric, the McKinsey consulting company, and Shell Oil.[1] Depending on whether a product or business falls in one of three areas, the strategic decision should be to either invest and *build* a position, balance cash flow to *hold* a position, or throw off cash to *harvest* a position. These options are displayed in Figure B–1.

---

[1] Michael E. Porter. *Competitive Strategy: Techniques for Analyzing Industries and Competitors* (New York: The Free Press, 1980). This review is based on 365–367.

Figure B–1.   Company Position/Industry Attractiveness Matrix

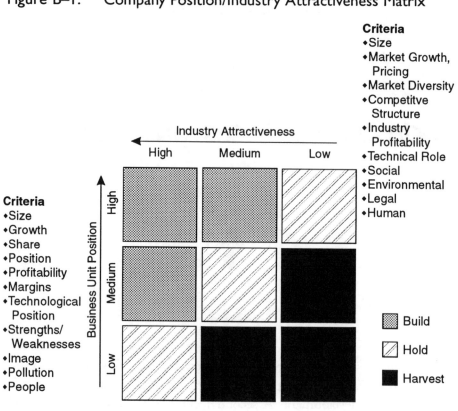

Criteria
◆Size
◆Market Growth,
   Pricing
◆Market Diversity
◆Competitve
   Structure
◆Industry
   Profitability
◆Technical Role
◆Social
◆Environmental
◆Legal
◆Human

Criteria
◆Size
◆Growth
◆Share
◆Position
◆Profitability
◆Margins
◆Technological
   Position
◆Strengths/
   Weaknesses
◆Image
◆Pollution
◆People

Industry Attractiveness

High   Medium   Low

Business Unit Position

High   Medium   Low

▨ Build

▨ Hold

■ Harvest

Source: Reprinted with the permission of The Free Press, a Division of Simon & Schuster from *Competitive Strategy: Techniques for Analyzing Industries and Competitors* by Michael E. Porter. Copyright © 1980 by The Free Press.

Another matrix that can be useful in strategy development relates a business organization's life cycle to the marketplace's life cycle. Hillestad and Berkowitz refer to this matrix as the strategy action match matrix, shown in Figure B–2.

With the strategy action match matrix, different configurations of the two life cycles suggest different strategies:[2]

---

[2] Steven Hillestad and Eric Berkowitz. *Healthcare Marketing Plans: From Strategy to Action* (Maryland: Aspen, 1991), 121–145. With the exception of a few modifications, the review below is taken entirely from the authors.

Figure B–2.   Strategy Action Match Matrix

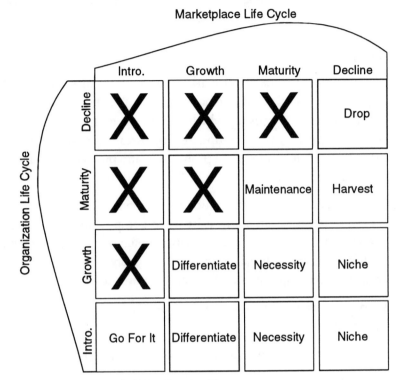

X = Position Cannot Occur

Source: Reprinted from Steven Hillestad and Eric Berkowitz. *Healthcare Marketing Plans* (Gaithersburg, Maryland: Aspen, 1991). Copyright © 1991 Aspen Publishers, Inc.

❑ **Go-for-it.** Both a business and a market are in introductory stages. Elements of a go-for-it strategy include establishing leadership and brand identity early, limiting product or service variations, emphasizing quality, pricing either higher for image or lower for market share, and creating entry barriers wherever possible.

❑ **Differentiation.** Business is in its introductory or growth stage, but the market is already in a growth stage. As the authors put it, "The later a business enters the market relative to the competition, the more difficult and expensive it becomes to establish a differential advantage." Consequently, "all the elements of the marketing mix"—product, price, place, and promotion—should be used to achieve effective differentiation.

❏ **Necessity.** Business introduces a new product to compete in an established market. A specialty clinic adding primary care providers when there is already an oversupply, or a traditional health insurer introducing a new HMO when the market is mature—both actions exemplify a necessity strategy.

❏ **Maintenance.** Business and market are in the mature stages of their respective life cycles. Maintenance calls for tactics that refine the marketing mix: Choosing which customers to serve or not serve, aggressive pricing to shore up existing customer relations, selective innovations, not letting up on promotion, and protecting distribution channels at all costs.

❏ **Niche.** Business is in an introductory or growth stage, but the market is declining. Niche situations exist when competitors have exited the market, but particular market segments remain stable. Successful niche strategies require minimal competition, accuracy in market projections and, as Porter emphasized, efficiencies to lower costs.

❏ **Harvest.** Business is in its mature phase, but the marketplace is declining.

❏ **Drop.** Business and the marketplace are both in declining phases.

Like the other techniques, the strength of this technique is that it ties specific strategies to specific circumstances. But like other techniques also, it runs the risk of being too absolute. In Hillestad's and Berkowitz's case, for example, niche strategies can be successfully pursued during growth or mature phases of a market's life cycle and need not be limited to the declining phase. In addition, if a management has the presence of mind to adjust, differentiation strategies can be pursued by start-up as well as established businesses at just about any phase in a market's life cycle. Finally, it is not unheard of for companies to be deliberate followers in growing markets and by design adopt a go-for-it strategy after others have already tested the waters and become fairly well established.

With that said, the product portfolio method pioneered by Henderson plus the two reviewed here are all useful tools to help management identify an overall business strategy.

APPENDIX C

Stakeholder Analysis and Strategy

Stakeholders cover the spectrum of society and come in a variety of organized and unorganized forms. In the current debate over national health policy, the national Chamber Commerce is considered a powerful stakeholder, but so too are organizations that represent the uninsured. While industry structure and the marketplace dictate the lion's share of what gets considered in strategy development, political factors associated with key stakeholders should not be discounted. It's not uncommon for an HMO to avoid some initiative because of political fallout from its provider panel or for a hospital to scratch a new innovation because it alienates some on the medical staff or for a business coalition to avoid working with a single source health vendor because it will antagonize other vendors tied to specific coalition members.

Nutt and Backoff have developed a series of matrices that help to analyze stakeholder issues in strategic thinking.[1] The first, presented in Figure C–1, represents a straightforward method for identifying four kinds of stakeholders.

Figure C–1.   Stakeholder Assessments

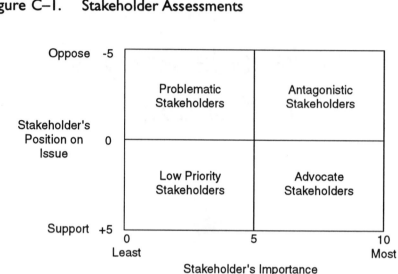

Source: Reprinted from Paul Nutt and Robert Backoff. *Strategic Management of Public and Third Sector Organizations* (San Francisco: Josey-Bass, 1992).

Knowing which stakeholders are a threat and which are not, who is important and who is not, can make a huge difference in the ultimate success of any business strategy.

Nutt and Backoff's second matrix, Figure C–2, enables organizations to categorize the kinds of resources that could be available to support a strategy, as well as their relative importance. No strategy can be successful if the resources needed for implementation are either unavailable or unlikely to be consistently available.

---

1 Paul Nutt and Robert Backoff. *Strategic Management of Public and Third Sector Organizations* (San Francisco: Josey Bass, 1992). My summaries are drawn from the authors' own comments in and around the pages where their figures appeared.

Figure C–2.   Resource Assessments

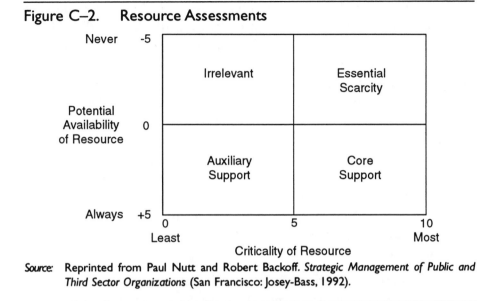

Source: Reprinted from Paul Nutt and Robert Backoff. *Strategic Management of Public and Third Sector Organizations* (San Francisco: Josey-Bass, 1992).

Where the first two methods reflect a snapshot of key stakeholder issues, a third matrix, Figure C–3, offers a more dynamic view, extending beyond stakeholder activity to an organization's ability to gain control over the whole gamut of political variables in its environment.

Figure C–3.   Types of Organizations

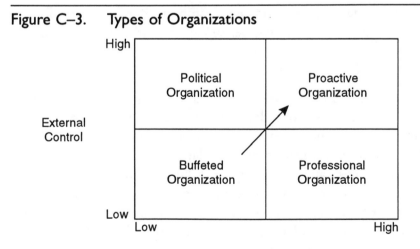

Source: Reprinted from Paul Nutt and Robert Backoff. *Strategic Management of Public and Third Sector Organizations* (San Francisco: Josey-Bass, 1992).

Paralleling the logic of product portfolio analysis, but from the standpoint of the political marketplace, Nutt and Backoff's matrix suggests three points about organizations that help to inform strategy development. First, there are four basic organization types, though two types—political and professional organizations—are by nature precluded from exercising effective control over their internal or external environment. Second, in the same way that cash cows are supposed to evolve to build stars out of question marks, successful strategy requires that buffeted organizations evolve towards proactive organizations. Finally, proactive organizations are distinguished by at least four core factors: 1) having a clear agenda tied to a generally acceptable vision; 2) incorporating important stakeholders, even those who disagree, into the process; 3) operating in a win-win context through cooperation rather than internal competition; and 4) always maintaining political and public support.

The issues portfolio matrix rounds out this stakeholder section. Portfolio analysis can be used by management to assess not just the impact of public and community issues on a business' strategy, but the impact of customer, supplier, and distributor issues on business strategy as well.

Nutt and Backoff categorize issues by how they stack up against two variables: Tractability and relative stakeholder support. Tractability they define as "The prospect that an issue can be attacked by an organization." Issues with high tractability are either going to be very important or are potentially very important. Issues with low stakeholder support are either not likely to gain very much acceptance or, for all intents and purposes, likely to remain dormant. Figure C–4 identifies four possible issue categories.

While it's not necessarily the case that business strategy should focus exclusively on issues that are sitting ducks, ignoring them will create misalignments that may well have negative consequences down the road. Brand name pharmaceutical companies ignoring the managed care industry's concern about rising costs and then scurrying at the 11th hour to spend billions to buy pharmacy benefit plans is one example.[2] Ultimately, successful business strategy requires some productive links to stakeholder concerns. This means that strategy should either reflect issues that are sitting ducks or

---

[2] See, for example, Milt Freudenheim. "A Shift of Power in Pharmaceuticals." *New York Times* (May 5, 1994): D1.

Figure C–4.   Issue Portfolio

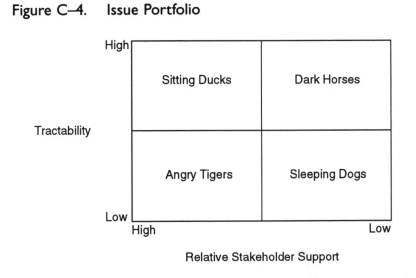

Relative Stakeholder Support

Source: Reprinted from Paul Nutt and Robert Backoff. *Strategic Management of Public and Third Sector Organizations* (San Francisco: Josey-Bass, 1992).

should reflect issues management intends to make sitting ducks—by increasing stakeholder support for dark horse issues or developing internal capacity to support angry tiger issues.

Glossary

Actuarial. Actuarial refers to risk and probability regarding illness and the utilization of health services. In healthcare generally, insurance companies make actuarial projections to set premiums and fee schedules; in HMOs, actuarial projections determine the capitation for specific kinds of providers.

Benefit Design. All health insurance plans have a benefit design. The benefit design defines an individual's health insurance coverage. On average, the more generous the benefit design, the more insurers will pay for health services.

Capitation. Capitation is a form of provider reimbursement used by HMOs expressed on a per-member per-month (pmpm) basis. Because HMOs require members to utilize a fixed panel of providers, they are able to project pmpm amounts that can then be assigned to specific providers. Primary care physicians are often capitated by HMOs; hospitals are sometimes capitated; and specialists as well as ancillary providers are occasionally capitated. Once providers are capitated, they are "at risk." This shifting of risk eliminates the perverse incentive under fee-for-service reimbursement for providers to overtreat patients, which is a central element in HMOs' unique cost-containment capability.

Case Rates. A case rate is bundled or all-inclusive payment for an entire patient episode, usually including physician and facility costs. Hospitals establish case rate arrangements with HMOs and PPOs for a variety of standard as well as tertiary surgical procedures. Not unlike capitation, case rates shift the risk in health insurance away from the payor under open-ended fee-for-service reimbursement, and place the provider at risk.

Center of Excellence. Centers of excellence are usually medical centers that excel in treating certain kinds of serious illnesses or performing specific tertiary surgical procedures. HMOs and PPOs enter into center-of-excellence relationships with selected providers both for quality reasons and to obtain discounts in exchange for patient channeling. Patients value these relationships because they know they are being sent to a leading physician and hospital for their particular health problem.

Contracting. Providers as well as managed care systems engage in contracting, but for different reasons. Provider contracting is an entrepreneurial activity. Laboratories, specialty networks, and primary care as well as multispecialty groups all are heavily involved in contracting, ideally, to obtain an exclusive franchise for delivering designated services to HMOs and PPOs. When managed care systems engage in contracting, it is as a necessary corporate function. Contracting in this context is part of everyday operations because it builds and maintains an HMO's or PPO's actual delivery system.

DRGs (Diagnostic-Related Groups). DRGs are a classification system enabling inpatient hospital stays to be assigned to a specific category for purposes of payment. The Healthcare Financing Administration (HCFA) originally developed this system for reimbursing Medicare patients' hospital stays, but DRGs are now used by private insurers as well as some individual states for all payors. Since length of stay, service intensity, and average cost of services are built into the payment associated with each of the over 470 DRGs, when a patient's length of stay is longer or a hospital's cost structure is higher than reflected in a specific DRG, hospitals lose money. Conversely, if length of stay is shorter and a hospital's cost structure is lower, hospitals make money.

ERISA. ERISA is an acronym for the Employee Retirement Income Security Act of 1974, which includes provisions for businesses to self-insure. Usually, businesses will not self-insure unless they have a minumum of 500 employees. Self-insured companies establish their own benefit design and assume the risk health insurers are ordinarily responsible for. In assuming risk, a company sets aside X amount of dollars to pay claims. Self-insured companies usually retain an HMO, PPO, and/or traditional health insurance carrier to administer their employees' health coverage—referred to as ASO or administrative only business. When a self-insured company offers its employees an HMO, in effect the HMO functions as an EPO.

Exclusive Provider Organization (EPO). EPOs are similar to both PPOs and HMOs in certain basic ways. Like PPOs, EPO providers are paid discount fee-for-service and are usually offered as an option by employers that self-insure. Like HMOs, the EPO benefit design limits members' access to those providers who participate with the health plan. Some EPOs also use a gatekeeper approach to regulate access to specialists.

Fee-for-Service. Fee-for-service is a form of reimbursement in which a fee is rendered for each service performed. Under fee-for-service, there is a perverse incentive for physicians to abuse the reimbursement process because the more frequent the patient visits and the more procedures a physician performs, the greater the physician's compensation. Where the "fee" used to almost always be based on physicians' charges, fee-for-service increasingly is defined by a discount fee schedule. California RVS, McGraw-Hill Relative Values For Physicians, and Medicare RBRVS are three of the most widely used discount fee schedules in the industry today.

Freedom of Choice. Like indemnity coverage, freedom of choice is a central element in traditional health insurance. It means that individuals may go to any physician or hospital they choose, and their health coverage will apply.

Health Maintenance Organization (HMO). HMOs are managed care systems that both insure *and* deliver health services to a covered population. HMOs are paid a premium like other health insurance carriers. Unlike traditional health insurers, though, they manage their premium dollar on a per-member per-month (pmpm) basis. This pmpm is referred to as a capitation. HMOs often capitate specific kinds of services, such as primary care and selected specialties. The benefit design for HMOs requires that members only use a set panel of providers, and that members incur a nominal co-payment for each physician visit. In some instances, HMOs are beginning to offer out-of-panel coverage as a benefit option for their members. Out-of-panel coverage is a plus from a marketing standpoint, but it makes it more difficult for management to project the pmpm amounts to be used when capitating physicians. There are many different kinds of HMOs. Three classic models are:

Staff. Physicians are employees of the HMO.

Group. The HMO capitates a separate medical group, and physicians in the group are compensated based on either salary, productivity, or some combination.

IPA. Physicians remain in their own private practices but contract on a "participating" basis with the HMO.

Currently, the trend is for HMOs to function as "health plans" and contract with separate provider-based fiduciary organizations. In addition to medical groups, the two organizations contracted with most frequently are:

IPAs comprised of physicians in private practice who contract directly with the IPA organization. Though there are exceptions—medical society sponsored IPAs in California, for example—these IPA HMOs represent the generation after direct-contract IPA model HMOs. They obtain a "professional only" capitation from the HMO healthplan.

Physician-Hospital Organizations (PHOs) are the product of a joint venture between a hospital, and interested members of the hospital medical staff who agree to participate in a physician organization (PO). PHOs obtain a professional *and* facility capitation from HMO health plans.

Indemnity. Indemnity health insurance is the classic form of fee-for-service, the original expression of the "property and casual" model of insurance in healthcare. Typically, under indemnity coverage 1) the physician charges whatever is deemed appropriate; 2) the patient pays the physician; and 3) after a deductible, the insurance carrier indemnifies the patient 80 percent of the physician's charge. Indemnity coverage established the foundation for healthcare inflation in the United States.

Managed Care. Managed care has two connotations. First, it is a term that gained wide use in the 1980s to describe any number of organized efforts to achieve cost containment in healthcare delivery. In this sense it refers to 1) alternative delivery systems such as HMOs and PPOs; 2) specific financial incentives that encourage individuals to use less-expensive providers such as preferred providers and outpatient surgery centers; and 3) nonindemnity forms of provider reimbursement, such as capitation, DRGs, case rates, and discount fee-for-service. Second, managed care refers to the period of healthcare industry evolution beyond the period characterized by solo practice, fee-for-service medicine.

Managed Care Systems. Managed care systems (referred to in the 1980s as alternative delivery systems) are organized arrangements of providers that deliver health services in accordance with stipulated benefit designs. Such systems include HMOs, PPOs, POS plans, and traditional indemnity health insurance coupled with preauthorization provisions. "Managed care plans" are synonymous with "managed care systems."

Managed Competition. Managed competition refers to a school of thought in health policy that embraces managed care as the key to healthcare reform. The principal goal of managed competition is to restructure the medical marketplace so it becomes more competitive, by changing the underlying organization of healthcare delivery from solo practitioners in an open-ended fee-for-service insurance environment, to physicians and hospitals operating in managed care systems.

Management Service Organizations (MSOs). MSOs provide information systems and administrative support to physician practices, medical groups, IPAs, PHOs, and various provider networks. MSO functions related to physician practices include billing, accounting, purchasing, payroll, obtaining malpractice insurance, employee leasing, and contracting. MSO functions for IPAs, PHOs, and provider networks include claims processing, utilization review, management reporting, provider profiling, provider relations, and contracting.

Networks. Networks are groups of providers (e.g., chiropractic networks, ophthalmology networks, hospital networks) that have usually been established to obtain exclusive agreements with HMOs or PPOs. Networks exist to contract with managed care plans. When physician networks operate in an HMO context, reimbursement is often on a capitation basis; in a PPO context, reimbursement is on a discount fee-for-service basis.

Panel/Out-of-Panel. Panels refer to physicians, hospitals, and other providers comprising an HMO or PPO. Out-of-panel refers to nonparticipating providers.

Participating (Par) Providers. Par providers participate in HMOs and PPOs. Participation is defined in a legal contract stipulating the provider's obligation to conform to various administrative, operational, financial, and clinical requirements of a managed care plan.

Perverse Incentive. Perverse incentives refer to financial biases associated with different forms of reimbursement that induce providers to render clinical decisions in less than a totally objective and professional way. Under fee-for-service, the perverse incentive is to do more than necessary to increase the provider's payment. Under capitation, the perverse incentive is to do less than necessary to reduce the provider's costs.

Point-of-Service (POS). POS plans are HMOs, usually with primary care physician/gatekeepers that provide out-of-panel coverage. POS plans represent the HMO industry's response to PPOs. By incorporating a POS component into HMOs, the assumption is that HMO market share will increase.

Preferred Provider Organization (PPO). PPOs are managed care systems that pay for health services members receive from participating providers. Like HMOs, members incur a nominal co-payment when they use a preferred provider. Unlike HMOs, PPOs are only able to reimburse their providers on a discount fee-for-service basis. By definition, PPOs offer out-of-panel coverage as an intrinsic feature of the health benefit. Usually, out-of-panel coverage takes effect after the member has met a deductible with coverage set between 70 and 80 percent of what the PPO defines as a reasonable charge. Out-of-panel PPO coverage is an indemnity benefit.

PPOs are sold by insurance companies as an "insured" product. However, they also operate in the large group market, (e.g., 500 employees or more) where employers self-insure. When employers self-insure, they "rent" a network and pay for all the utilization review and claims processing administration the health benefit requires. In the insurance industry, this is referred to as "administrative services only" or ASO business. Since ASO arrangements place the employer, not the insurer, at risk, employers purchase re-insurance to protect for loses above a stipulated amount. Commercial health insurance companies and Blue Cross Plans offer ASO business along with their insured products.

Prepaid. Prepaid is payment rendered in advance of the actual delivery of health services. Capitation represents prepaid healthcare. Prepaid arrangements place providers at risk.

Primary Care Physicians (PCPs). PCPs are physicians whose expertise is not limited to one body system or type of disease such as eyes, heart, bone, or cancer. Family practitioners, internists, and pediatricians are PCPs. In many instances, the primary care label also extends to obstetrics-gynecology. HMOs have made the PCP role central to patient management. Currently, most HMOs require their members to have a designated PCP. The PCP is responsible for providing certain preventive services and the full spectrum of primary care, as well as making the formal referral to specialists. Usually, without an explicit PCP referral, specialty coverage is denied by HMOs. Regulating access to specialists by PCPs is called the "gatekeeper" function. Gatekeepers are only occasionally used by PPOs and do not exist when health insurance is governed by freedom of choice (e.g., Medicare).

Utilization Management. Utilization management encompasses utilization review as well as various clinical management and reporting functions designed to monitor physician performance and improve quality of care. In addition to traditional utilization review, utilization management includes physician profiling, outcomes research, and use of clinical protocols to standardize physicians' decision making.

Utilization Review (UR). UR refers to different administrative procedures employed by the insurer to control patients' use of medical services and providers' use of medical resources. UR includes 1) preauthorization, 2) concurrent review, 3) retrospective review, and 4) catastrophic case management. UR exists in PPOs but is especially prominent in HMOs. The preauthorization component of UR has become almost a standard feature in traditional indemnity health insurance.

Index